NLN
PRESS

NURSE EDUCATORS 1997

Findings from the RN and LPN Faculty Census

JONES AND BARTLETT PUBLISHERS

Sudbury, Massachusetts

BOSTON   TORONTO   LONDON   SINGAPORE

World Headquarters

Jones and Bartlett Publishers
40 Tall Pine Drive
Sudbury, MA 01776
978-443-5000
info@jbpub.com
www.jbpub.com

Jones and Bartlett Publishers Canada
P.O. Box 19020
Toronto, ON M5S 1X1
CANADA

Jones and Bartlett Publishers International
Barb House, Barb Mews
London W6 7PA
UK

Copyright © 1999 by Jones and Bartlett Publishers, Inc. and National League for Nursing

ISBN: 0-7637-1011-3

Printed in the United States of America
02 01 00 99 98   10 9 8 7 6 5 4 3 2 1

PREFACE

The National League for Nursing's Division of Research presents the new **Nurse Educators 1997: Findings from the Faculty Census**—a compilation of findings of NLN's biennial study of nursing faculty for all RN, LPN, and higher educational programs.

Like all publications from NLN Research, the tables, graphs, and detailed explanation of data will prove to be a valuable resource for your own research needs. The data presented here is especially pertinent for all of us to review and analyze carefully as nursing education is transformed to match the changing face of health care. Important to note in these findings is the increased ration of part-time to full-time faculty across all nursing education programs, especially in baccalaureate programs, as well as an increase in faculty salaries.

The following Executive Summary highlights the trends that are emerging in this already changing system of care, explains the reasons for these trends, and anticipates what we can expect in the future. The pages of tables, graphs, and charts clearly expand upon this general analysis for further understanding and extrapolation of data.

NLN Research has continued to grow and expand to match a profession whose needs are many and whose future is invaluable to healthy communities. I am sure you will agree as you discover the wealth of information provided in **Nurse Educators 1997: Findings from the Faculty Census.**

Delroy Louden, PhD
Vice President
NLN Research

CONTENTS

DEFINITION OF TERMS

Administrator of Nursing Program—Dean, chair, director, head of department

Baccalaureate Programs

a) *Baccalaureate and higher degree programs:* All baccalaureate and graduate nursing programs

b) *Baccalaureate and higher degree programs with basic students:* Programs that accept students without prior nursing education. Most of these programs also admit registered nurses who had previously studied at the associate degree or diploma level and are returning to baccalaureate nursing education. Master's and doctoral level programs are also included with these programs.

c) *Baccalaureate and higher degree programs with non-basic students (for RN students only)*: Programs designed exclusively for registered nurses returning for baccalaureate education (BRN programs) and/or graduate education.

Ethnic Background—The categories used to denote ethnic background are:

a) American Indian or Alaskan Native
b) Asian or Pacific Islander
c) Black, Non-Hispanic
d) Hispanic
e) White, Non-Hispanic

FTE—Full-time equivalents are calculated by assuming each part-time faculty member is equivalent to one-half of a full-time faculty member.

Full-time Nurse Faculty—Individuals contracted on a full-time basis to teach or supervise students.

Highest Earned Credential—The highest earned degree or diploma held by a faculty member.

Non-Nurse Faculty—Individuals who are not registered nurses and are contracted to teach students as a part of the nursing faculty.

Salary

a) Academic Year Salary: Salary based on a nine-month work year.

b) Calendar Year Salary: Salary based on a twelve-month work year.

Part-time Nurse Faculty—Individuals employed less than the required hours for a full-time faculty employment.

Unfilled Positions—Full-time budgeted positions not filled as of January 1994.

Vacancy Rate—Budgeted vacancies/Total Full-Time Positions and Budgeted Vacancies.

JURISDICTIONS INCLUDED IN THE NLN REGIONS

North Atlantic	**Midwestern**	**Southern**	**Western**
Connecticut	Illinois	Alabama	Alaska
Delaware	Indiana	Arkansas	Arizona
District of Columbia	Iowa	Florida	California
Maine	Kansas	Georgia	Colorado
Massachusetts	Michigan	Kentucky	Hawaii
New Hampshire	Minnesota	Louisiana	Idaho
New Jersey	Missouri	Maryland	Montana
New York	Nebraska	Mississippi	Nevada
Pennsylvania	North Dakota	North Carolina	New Mexico
Rhode Island	Ohio	Oklahoma	Oregon
Vermont	South Dakota	South Carolina	Utah
	Wisconsin	Tennessee	Washington
		Texas	Wyoming
		Virginia	
		West Virginia	

Section 1
Executive Summary

EXECUTIVE SUMMARY

TOTAL ESTIMATED FACULTY

Overall, the total estimated number of nurse faculty increased by 3.7 percent between 1994 and 1996, with full-time faculty increasing by 2.7 percent, part-time faculty increasing by 7.6 percent, and unfilled budgeted positions increasing by three percent (Figure 1). The percentage increase in estimated full-time faculty was similar to the increase experienced between 1992 and 1994. In contrast, the percentage increase for part-time faculty was not as great as in previous years where the increases ranged from 14 percent to 29 percent.

The changes in the estimated number of nursing faculty varied considerably by program type. For baccalaureate and higher degree programs, total estimated faculty increased by 5.1 percent, with full-time faculty increasing by just 2.1 percent, while part-time faculty increased by 18.1 percent. In contrast, total estimated faculty in diploma programs decreased by 22.7 percent, with full-time faculty decreasing by 20.8 percent and part-time faculty decreasing by 33.4 percent. Associate degree programs remained relatively stable with a nominal decrease of 0.3 percent in total estimated faculty; full-time faculty increased by less than one percent, and part-time faculty decreased by four percent. Estimated unfilled budgeted positions also varied by program type, with positions at associate degree programs increasing by 21.4 percent, while positions in diploma and baccalaureate and higher degree programs decreased by 17.9 percent and 11.3 percent, respectively.

AVERAGE NUMBER OF FACULTY

In 1996, the overall average (mean) number of full-time and part-time faculty were almost identical to the averages in 1994. Program types were examined using matched pair t-test comparisons for schools which responded both in 1994 and in 1996. According to the results, there was a significant increase in the mean number of full-time and part-time baccalaureate and higher degree faculty, a significant decrease in the mean number of part-time associate degree faculty, and a significant decrease in the mean number of full-time and part-time diploma faculty (See Table 1a). There were no significant changes in the number of practical/vocational nursing faculty.

When the overall mean number of faculty were compared for all schools which responded in 1994 or in 1996, without the requirement of matched pairs, the mean number of full-time faculty in baccalaureate and higher degree programs dropped from 19.7 in 1994 to 16.9 in 1996 (Figure 2). For Diploma programs, the mean number of full-time faculty dropped from 13.8 to 11.8 and the mean number of part-time faculty dropped from 4.5 to 3.3. There were nominal changes for associate degree and practical/vocational nursing programs. These overall means indicate the average number of faculty for nursing education programs in 1994 and in 1996. The matched pair results indicate the direction of change in the average number of faculty within the schools of nursing.

The overall vacancy rate also increased from 4.4 in 1994 to 4.8 in 1996 (Figure 3). Increased vacancy rates occurred across program type, with the exception of baccalaureate and higher degree programs where it dropped from 5.7 to 5.0. The greatest increase occurred in practical/vocational nursing programs, from 2.8 to 5.6, between 1994 and 1996.

PRIMARY TEACHING RESPONSIBILITY

Primary teaching responsibility for nursing faculty was examined according to highest earned credential. As would be expected, full-time nursing faculty who had doctorates as the highest earned credential primarily taught baccalaureate (49.2%) or graduate courses (40.7%). Approximately 45 percent of nursing faculty with masters' degrees primarily taught associate degree courses, although 34.4 percent reported baccalaureate programs as their primary teaching responsibility (Figure 4). The majority of nursing faculty with baccalaureate degrees taught in practical/vocational programs (66.1%), with an additional 25.4 percent primarily teaching in associate degree programs. The great majority of nurse faculty with other nursing credentials primarily taught in practical/vocational nursing programs (91.6%), with an additional 4.9 percent who primarily taught in associate degree programs.

RACIAL AND ETHNIC BACKGROUND

There were nominal increases in the racial/ethnic diversity of nursing education administrators, growing from 8.5 percent to 9.7 percent. As in 1994, the greatest diversity was in the West, with 88.6 percent white; 3.1 percent Hispanic; 2.6 percent black; 4.8 percent Asian/Pacific Islander; and 0.9 percent American Indian/Alaskan Native. With respect to program type, practical/vocational nursing programs had the greatest diversity, with the least diversity found in Diploma programs (Figure 5).

The racial/ethnic background of full-time faculty experienced very little change between 1994 and 1996 as well, with the percentage of minority faculty going from 9.5 percent to 9.1 percent of full-time faculty. As with the nursing administrators, the greatest diversity was found in the West, with 87.2 percent white; 2.8 percent Hispanic; 4.4 percent black; 4.8 percent Asian/Pacific Islander; and 0.8 percent American Indian/Alaskan Native. With respect to program type, practical/vocational nursing programs had the greatest diversity, and Baccalaureate and Higher Degree Programs had the least diversity (Figure 6).

NURSE AND NON-NURSE FACULTY

Overall, only 2.1 percent of nursing school faculty were non-nurses. This varied by program type, with less than two percent teaching in associate degree and baccalaureate and higher degree programs; 3.4 percent in practical/vocational nursing programs; and 6.6 percent in diploma programs (Figure 7). In addition, a higher percentage of part-time faculty, 5.4 percent, were non-nurses. This also varied by program type, ranging from 2.5 percent in associate degree programs to 11.9 percent in diploma programs.

HIGHEST EARNED CREDENTIAL

With respect to nursing education administrators, there was an increase in the percentage with doctorates, as compared to master's degrees or other credentials, growing from 31.6 percent in 1994 to 41.1 percent in 1996. With respect to program type, the overwhelming majority of administrators for baccalaureate and higher degree programs, 92.3 percent, had doctorates while the majority of administrators for associate degree, diploma and practical/vocational nursing programs had master's degrees as the highest earned credential (Figure 8).

With respect to full-time faculty, there was a nominal increase in the percentage with doctorates, growing from 21.2 percent in 1994 to 24.7 percent in 1996. The percentage with master's degrees remained stable, going from 62 to 63 percent, while the percentage with baccalaureate degrees declined from 12.8 to 9.6 percent. With respect to program type, 46.1 percent of the full-time faculty at baccalaureate and higher degree programs had doctorates, and just over 50 percent had master's degrees as the highest earned credential (Figure 9). The overwhelming majority of associate degree and diploma faculty, over 85 percent, had master's degrees as the highest earned credential. The highest percentage of full-time practical/vocational nursing faculty had baccalaureate degrees (43.9%), and an additional 37.1 percent had master's degrees as the highest earned credential.

FACULTY RANK

Between 1994 and 1996, there was a higher percentage of professors, associate professors and assistant professors, with a lower percentage of instructors (Figure 10). In baccalaureate and higher degree programs, the percentage of professors increased from 9 percent to 10.5 percent, and the percentage of associate professors increased from 26.7 percent to 27.5 percent. The highest percentage of faculty, 40.1 percent, were assistant professors. In associate degree programs, the percentage of professors also increased, from 11.8 percent to 14.6 percent. The highest percentage of faculty, 37 percent, were instructors. Approximately 75 percent of diploma and practical/vocational nursing faculty held the rank of instructor.

SALARY

Overall, the highest percentage of administrators (39%) had a salary range of $45,000 to $59,999, with an additional 22.4 percent earning $30,000-$44,999, and 24.1 percent earning $60,000-$74,999. With respect to program type, 32.1 percent of administrators for baccalaureate and higher degree programs earned $75,000 or more, 32.2 percent earned $60,000 to $74,999, and 27.5 percent earned $45,000 to $59,999. The highest percentage of administrators for associate degree programs (48.5%) earned $45,000 to $59,999, with 23.5 percent earning $60,000 to $74,999 and 21.3 percent earning $30,000 to $44,999. The highest percentage of diploma administrators (48.6%) earned $60,000 to $74,999, and 18.6 percent earned $75,000 or more. Administrators for licensed practical/vocational nursing programs were equally distributed with 41.9 percent earning $45,000 to $59,999, and 40.9 percent earning $30,000 to $44,999.

Overall, the majority of full-time faculty (56.3%) earned $30,000 to $44,999, with 27.5% earning $45,000 to $59,999, and 9.3 percent earning $60,000 or more. With respect to program type, 51.7 percent of full-time faculty at baccalaureate and higher degree programs earned $30,000 to $44,999, with an additional 30.8 percent earning $45,000 to $59,999, and 14 percent earning $60,000 or more. As would be expected, there was considerable variation by faculty rank. Approximately 60 percent of professors earned $60,000 or more, 50 percent of associate professors earned $45,000 to $59,999, and the majority of assistant professors and instructors earned $30,000 to $44,999 (Figure 11).

With respect to associate degree programs, 61.3 percent of full-time faculty earned $30,000 to $44,999. In terms of faculty rank, approximately 40 percent of professors earned $45,000 to $59,999, with another 40 percent earning $30,000 to $44,999. The majority of associate professors, assistant professors and instructors earned $30,000 to $44,999 (Figure 12).

The majority of full-time diploma faculty earned $30,000 to $44,999, which was generally the case across faculty ranks as well (Figure 13). The majority of full-time faculty in practical/vocational nursing programs also earned $30,000 to $44,999, which was the case across faculty ranks, except for professors with approximately 15 percent earning $60,000 or more, and 49 percent earning $45,000 to $59,999 (Figure 14).

SALARY OF NURSING FACULTY COMPARED TO OTHER FACULTY MEMBERS

In April, 1997 the Chronicle of Higher Education reported the results from the College and University Personnel Association survey concerning annual salary for undergraduate faculty for the 1996-97 academic year.[1] According to the results, "At the bottom of the pay scale, the lowest-paid professors at public colleges are in nursing where the average salary this year is $42,966 ..." (P.13). By comparison, in 1996 the average annual salary for a nurse practitioner/midwife was $54,182, for a clinical nurse specialist it was $47,160, and for a certified nurse anesthetist it was $86,319 (Moses, 1997).[2] This salary differential occurs at a time when the growth in nursing education is at baccalaureate and higher degree levels, which require faculty who are prepared at the master's or doctoral level.[3,4] However, convincing nurses with advanced degrees to pursue a career in academia is particularly difficult when compared to salaries available in practice, and when compared to salaries of professors in all other academic departments.

In a recent article by Dr. Edward O'Neil (1997), executive director of the Pew Health Commission, he stated,

...nurses are in an excellent position to benefit from the transition to managed care. Not only do nurses practice in almost every imaginable health care setting, they possess valuable skills in case management, the psychosocial dimensions of health, and teamwork - all of which are being increasingly emphasized these days. (p. 4)

This statement indicates that nursing's important contributions to health care are being recognized by leaders in the health care field. Unfortunately, it appears that institutions of higher education do not recognize nor reward nursing's contribution within the academic setting.

Donna Post, PhD

Center for Research in Nursing
Education and Community Health

REFERENCES

1. Faculty salaries outpace inflation at public college, survey finds. (1997, April). The Chronicle of Higher Education, 43*(33), A12-A13.*

2. Moses, E.B. (1997). 1996 The registered nurse population: Findings from the National Sample Survey of Registered Nurses, March 1996. *Washington, DC: Division of Nursing, Bureau of Health Professions, Health Resources and Services Administration.*

3. Post, D., & Louden, D. (1997). Executive summary. Nursing DataSource 1997: Volume I-Trends in contemporary RN nursing education. *New York: National League for Nursing Press.*

4. Louden, D. (In press). Executive summary. Nursing DataSource 1997: Volume II-Graduate education in nursing advanced practice nursing. *New York: National League for Nursing Press.*

5. O'Neil, E. (1997). Trends to watch in health professions practice and education. Front & Center, 2*(2), pp. 4, 7.*

TABLE 1A. T-TESTS FOR PAIRED SAMPLES (MEAN NUMBER OF FACULTY)

BACCALAUREATE AND HIGHER DEGREE PROGRAMS

	YEAR		
	1994	1996	t-value
	(n=343)	(n=343)	(df=342)
FACULTY STATUS			
Full-time Faculty	18.7	19.6	4.00**
Part-time Faculty	8.8	10.5	4.38**
Total Faculty	27.5	30.0	5.99**

Associate Degree Programs	YEAR		
	1994	1996	t-value
	(n=604)	(n=604)	(df=603)
FACULTY STATUS			
Full-time Faculty	8.9	8.8	1.05
Part-time Faculty	5.7	5.3	2.77*
Total Faculty	14.7	14.2	2.75*

Diploma Programs	YEAR		
	1994	1996	t-value
	(n=84)	(n=84)	(df=83)
FACULTY STATUS			
Full-time Faculty	13.9	11.8	4.41**
Part-time Faculty	4.6	3.3	5.04**
Total Faculty	18.5	15.0	6.44**

Practical/Vocational Nursing Programs	YEAR		
	1994	1996	t-value
	(n=560)	(n=560)	(df=559)
FACULTY STATUS			
Full-time Faculty	3.9	4.0	1.19
Part-time Faculty	2.1	2.1	0.48
Total Faculty	6.0	6.1	0.56

Note: * $p < .05$ level, ** $p < .001$ level.

Section 2
Graphs

Figure 1

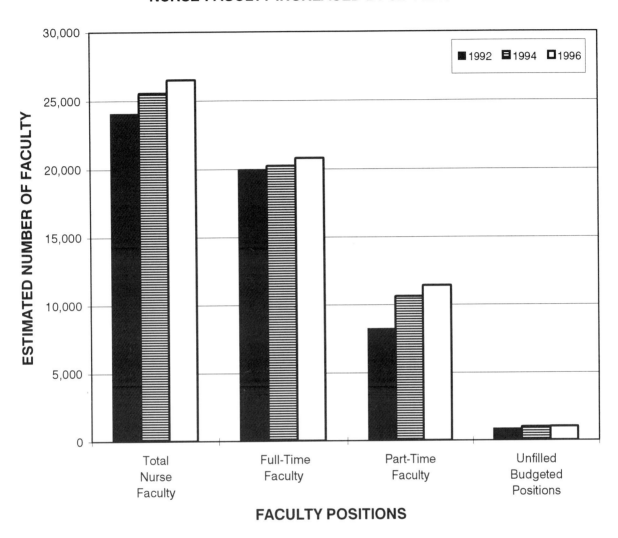

TOTAL ESTIMATED NUMBER OF
NURSE-FACULTY INCREASED BY 3.7 PERCENT

Figure 2

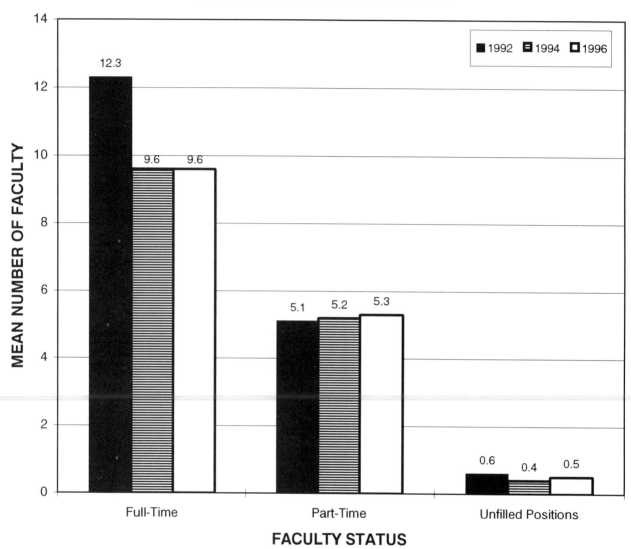

MEAN NUMBER OF FACULTY REMAINED
STABLE BETWEEN 1994 AND 1996

Figure 3

PN/VN PROGRAMS HAD GREATEST INCREASE IN VACANCY RATE

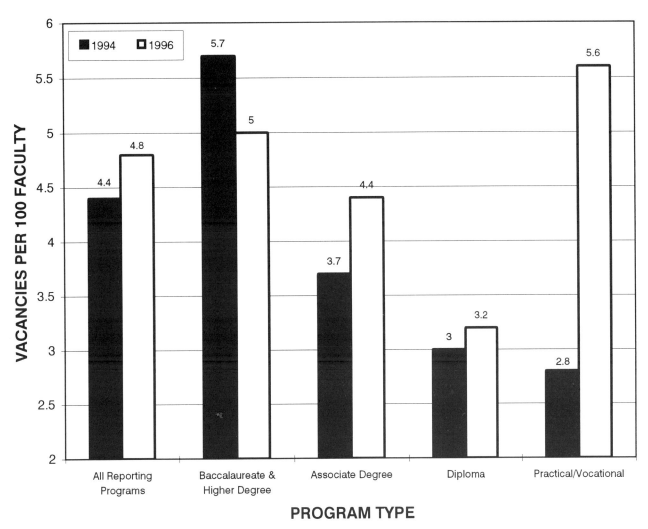

Figure 4

PRIMARY TEACHING RESPONSIBILITY OF FULL-TIME FACULTY BY HIGHEST EARNED CREDENTIAL

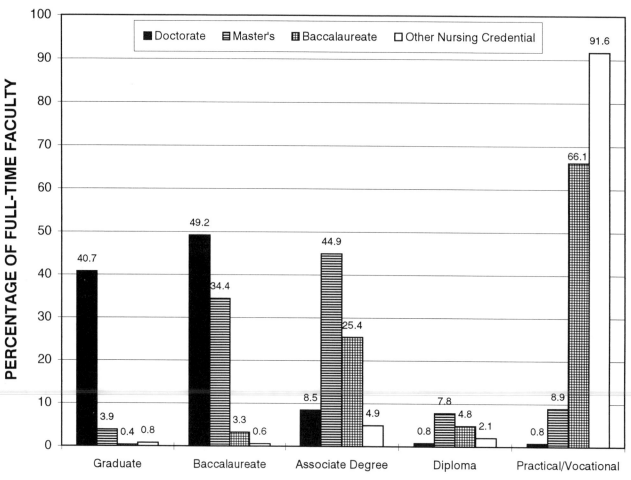

Figure 5

NURSING ADMINISTRATORS FOR PN/VN PROGRAMS
HAD GREATEST RACIAL/ETHNIC DIVERSITY

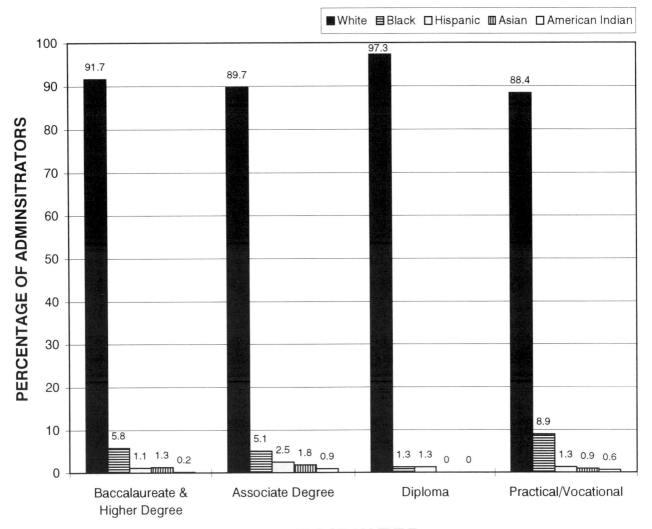

15

Figure 6

PRACTICAL/VOCATIONAL NURSING FULL-TIME
FACULTY HAD GREATEST RACIAL/ETHNIC DIVERSITY

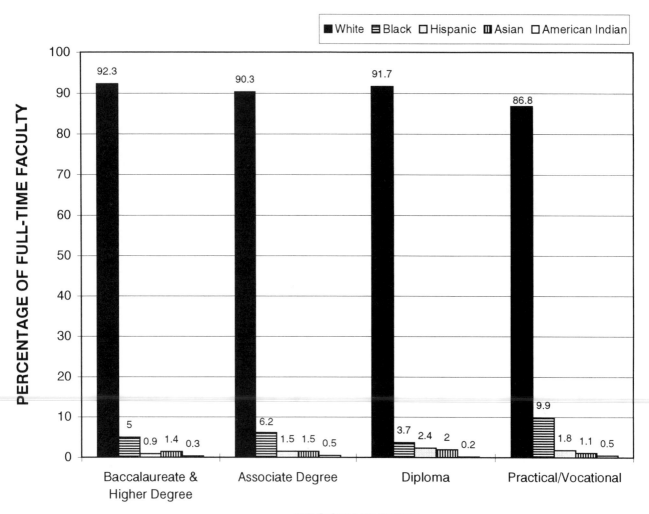

Figure 7

PERCENTAGE OF NON-NURSE FACULTY WAS HIGHER AMONG PART-TIME, AS COMPARED TO FULL-TIME FACULTY

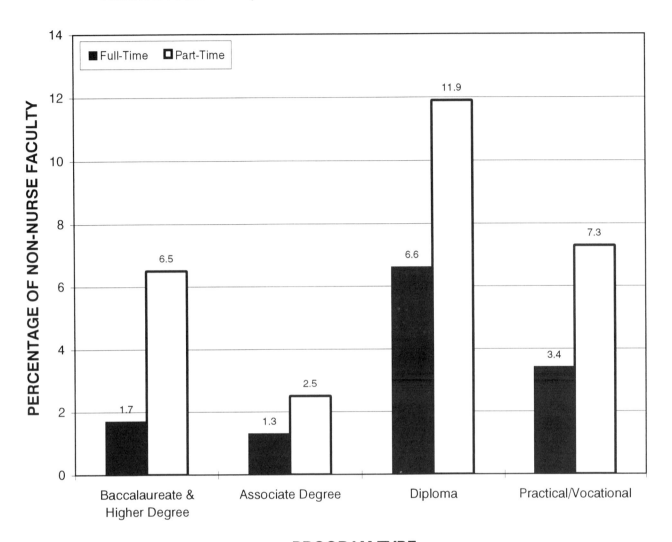

Figure 8

HIGHEST EARNED CREDENTIAL FOR NURSING EDUCATION ADMINISTRATORS VARIED BY PROGRAM TYPE

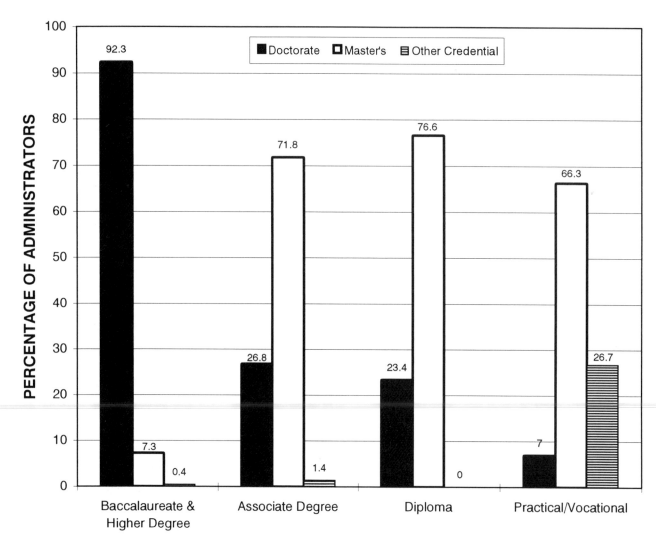

Figure 9

OVER 85% OF ASSOCIATE DEGREE AND DIPLOMA FULL-TIME FACULTY HAD MASTER'S AS HIGHEST EARNED CREDENTIAL

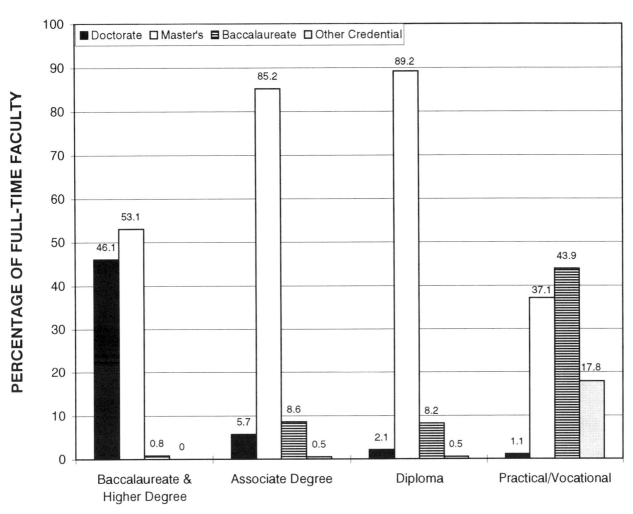

Figure 10

PERCENTAGE OF FULL-TIME INSTRUCTORS
DECLINED FROM 1994 TO 1996

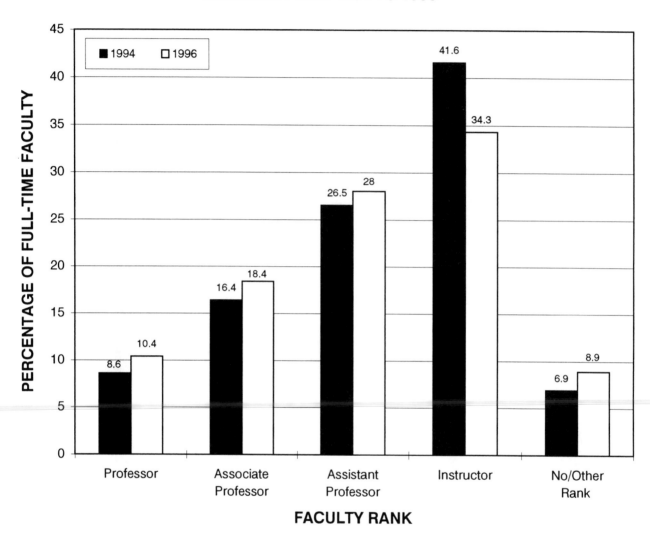

Figure 11

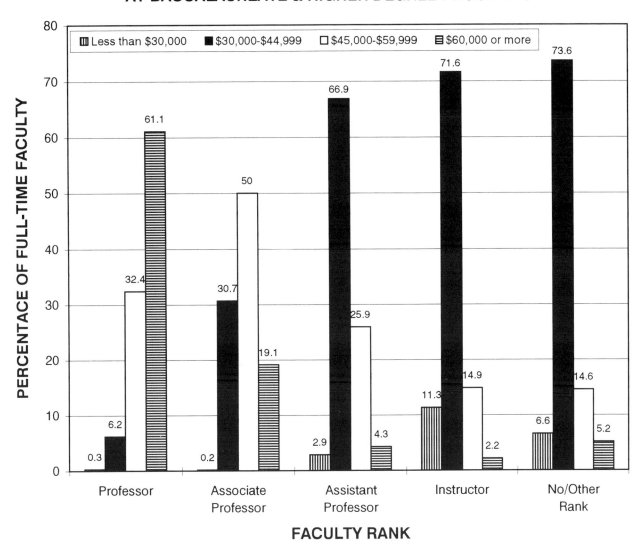

**SALARY RANGE FOR FULL-TIME FACULTY
AT BACCALAUREATE & HIGHER DEGREE PROGRAMS**

Figure 12

SALARY RANGE FOR FULL-TIME FACULTY
AT ASSOCIATE DEGREE PROGRAMS

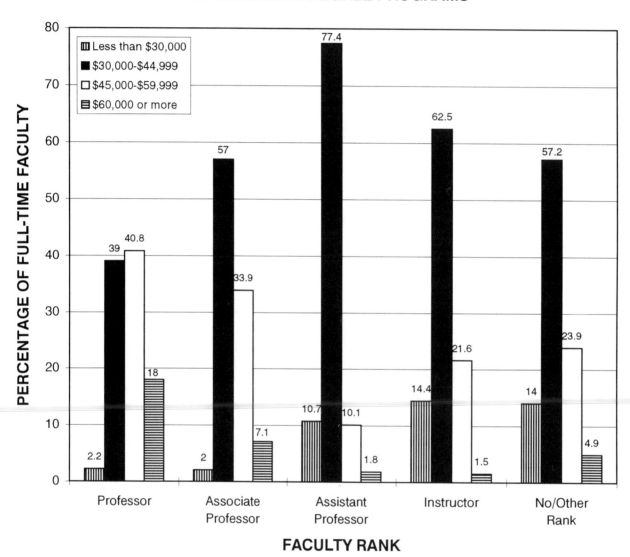

22

Figure 13

SALARY RANGE FOR FULL-TIME
FACULTY AT DIPLOMA PROGRAMS

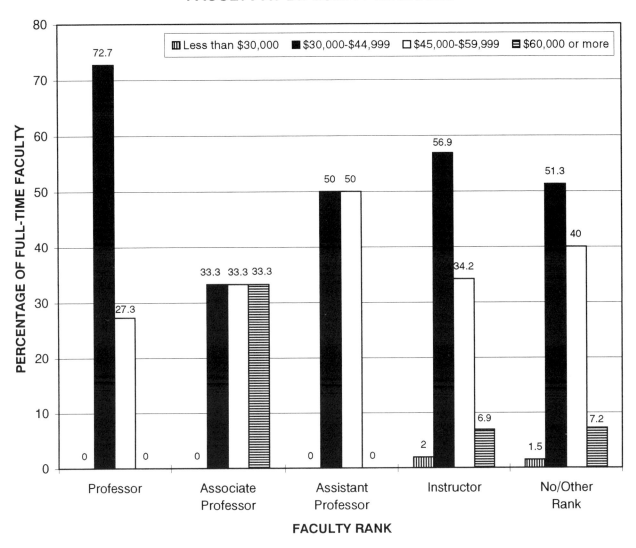

FACULTY RANK

Figure 14

SALARY RANGE FOR FULL-TIME FACULTY AT
PRACTICAL/VOCATIONAL NURSING PROGRAMS

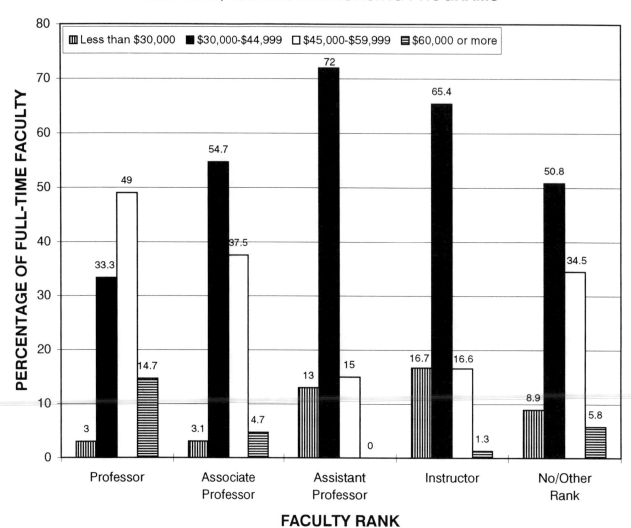

Section 3
Numeric Tables

NUMBER OF NURSING EDUCATION PROGRAMS BY STATE, REGION AND TYPE OF PROGRAM, 1996[1]

JURISDICTION	TOTAL NUMBER OF PROGRAMS	Diploma Programs	Associate Degree Programs	Baccalaureate and Higher Degree Programs		PN/VN Programs
				Basic Programs	Non-Basic Programs	
United States	2,767	119	876	521	144	1107
North Atlantic	560	63	153	115	53	176
Midwest	741	31	246	164	42	258
South	1,056	24	311	181	35	505
West	410	1	166	61	14	168
Alabama	59	0	23	13	1	22
Alaska	2	0	1	1	0	0
Arizona	31	0	13	4	1	13
Arkansas	50	2	11	9	0	28
California	172	1	71	24	7	69
Colorado	35	0	10	7	1	17
Connecticut	32	3	6	8	3	12
Delaware	12	1	4	2	2	3
District of Columbia	8	0	1	4	0	3
Florida	85	1	26	13	4	41
Georgia	76	0	20	13	5	38
Hawaii	11	0	4	3	0	4
Idaho	13	0	5	3	0	5
Illinois	115	4	42	27	6	36
Indiana	71	1	25	20	3	22
Iowa	71	5	25	12	3	26
Kansas	49	0	19	11	2	17
Kentucky	55	0	25	10	3	17
Louisiana	69	1	9	13	1	45
Maine	21	0	8	7	1	5
Maryland	36	2	14	7	2	11
Massachusetts	71	7	21	16	7	20
Michigan	78	2	32	15	2	27
Minnesota	49	0	12	9	4	24
Mississippi	39	0	16	7	1	15
Missouri	98	4	27	17	11	39
Montana	11	0	3	2	1	5
Nebraska	23	1	7	6	2	7
Nevada	8	0	4	2	0	2
New Hampshire	12	0	6	3	1	2
New Jersey	70	16	14	8	9	23
New Mexico	24	0	13	2	1	8
New York	168	5	63	32	14	54
North Carolina	95	3	47	12	2	31
North Dakota	14	0	0	7	1	6
Ohio	116	13	34	22	6	41
Oklahoma	59	0	17	11	1	30
Oregon	27	0	13	3	0	11
Pennsylvania	148	30	23	31	14	50
Rhode Island	8	1	3	3	0	1
South Carolina	45	0	13	8	1	23
South Dakota	13	0	6	4	1	2
Tennessee	64	4	14	18	2	26
Texas	186	2	49	26	5	104
Utah	14	0	4	3	1	6
Vermont	10	0	4	1	2	3
Virginia	94	8	17	12	4	53
Washington	48	0	18	6	2	22
West Virginia	44	1	10	9	3	21
Wisconsin	44	1	17	14	1	11
Wyoming	14	0	7	1	0	6
American Samoa	3	0	1	0	0	2
Guam	1	0	0	1	0	0
Puerto Rico	74	0	17	14	0	43
Virgin Islands	4	0	1	1	0	2

[1] Territories omitted from total.

Table 2
CHANGE IN NUMBER OF FULL-TIME AND PART-TIME FACULTY AND UNFILLED POSITIONS BY TYPE OF PROGRAM, 1986-1996[1,2]

NUMBER OF FACULTY AND UNFILLED BUDGETED POSITIONS BY TYPE OF PROGRAM[3]	1986		1988		1990		1992		1994		1996	
	Number	Percent Change	Number	Percent Change	Number	Percent Change	Number	Percent Change	Number	Percent Change	Number	Percent Change
ALL PROGRAMS REPORTING[4]												
Number of Programs Reporting	1,467	-5.7	1,451	-1.1	1,426	-1.7	1,366	-4.2	1,293	-5.3	1,342	+3.8
Percent of total programs	88.7	-3.6	88.4	-0.3	88.7	+0.3	84.4	-4.3	83.7	-0.7	80.8	-2.9
Number of full-time faculty	18,060	-11.7	16,813	-6.9	16,723	-0.5	16,836	+0.7	16,938	+0.6	16,800	-0.8
Number of part-time faculty	5,746	-9.1	5,372	-6.5	6,187	+15.2	6,939	+12.1	8,883	+28.0	9,225	+3.8
Unfilled budgeted positions	611	-12.0	768	+25.7	700	-8.8	726	+3.7	826	+13.8	821	-0.6
BACCALAUREATE AND HIGHER DEGREE PROGRAMS REPORTING[4]												
Number of Programs Reporting	557	-1.2	578	+3.8	547	-5.4	548	+0.2	433	-21.0	564	+30.2
Percent of total programs	91.2	+1.2	90.7	-0.5	85.7	-5.0	86.3	+0.6	77.6	-8.7	84.8	+7.2
Number of full-time faculty	8,925	-8.9	9,111	+0.2	8,615	-5.4	8,955	+3.9	8,524	-4.8	9,509	+11.6
Number of part-time faculty	2,845	+5.5	2,557	-10.1	2,605	+1.9	2,870	+10.2	3,979	+38.6	5,135	+29.0
Unfilled budgeted positions	402	-1.2	471	+17.2	402	-14.6	463	+15.2	513	+10.8	497	-3.1
ASSOCIATE DEGREE PROGRAMS REPORTING												
Number of Programs Reporting	692	-7.1	689	-0.4	730	+6.0	694	-4.9	744	+7.2	685	-7.9
Percent of total programs	87.9	-9.6	86.6	-1.3	89.9	+3.3	82.8	-7.1	86.8	+4.0	78.2	-8.6
Number of full-time faculty	6,288	-4.8	5,686	-9.6	6,254	+10.0	6,248	-0.1	6,814	+9.0	6,191	-9.1
Number of part-time faculty	2,395	-6.2	2,416	+0.9	3,156	+30.6	3,643	+15.4	4,380	+20.2	3,787	-13.5
Unfilled budgeted positions	138	-26.6	201	+45.7	206	+2.5	217	+5.3	263	+21.2	288	+9.5
DIPLOMA PROGRAMS REPORTING												
Number of Programs Reporting	218	-15.2	184	-15.6	149	-19.0	124	-16.8	116	+6.5	93	-19.8
Percent of total programs	85.2	-3.7	88.0	+2.8	94.9	+6.9	85.5	-9.4	89.9	+4.4	78.1	-11.8
Number of full-time faculty	2,847	-29.6	2,016	-29.2	1,854	-8.0	1,633	-11.9	1,600	-2.0	1,100	-31.2
Number of part-time faculty	506	-34.4	399	-21.1	426	+6.8	426	—	524	+23.0	303	-42.2
Unfilled budgeted positions	71	-28.3	96	+35.2	92	-4.2	46	-50.0	50	+8.7	36	-28.0

[1] As of January of each year indicated.
[2] Excludes American Samoa, Guam, Puerto Rico and the Virgin Islands.
[3] Directors of programs not included in table.
[4] Includes master's programs and RN baccalaurate programs.

Table 3
ESTIMATED NUMBER OF FULL-TIME AND PART-TIME FACULTY AND UNFILLED POSITIONS AND PERCENT CHANGE BY TYPE OF PROGRAM, 1986-1996[1,2]

ESTIMATED TOTAL NUMBER OF NURSE FACULTY AND UNFILLED BUDGETED POSITIONS BY TYPE OF PROGRAM[3]	1986		1988		1990		1992		1994		1996	
	Number	Percent Change	Number	Percent Change	Number	Percent Change	Number	Percent Change	Number	Percent Change	Number	Percent Change
ALL PROGRAMS[4]												
Total Number of Programs	1,654	-2.5	1,642	-0.7	1,607	-2.1	1,618	+0.7	1,544	-4.6	1,660	+7.5
Total estimated nurse-faculty (full-time and FTEs)[5]	23,600	-7.7	22,058	-6.5	22,341	+1.3	24,059	+7.7	25,531	+6.1	26,488	+3.7
Total estimated full-time faculty	20,361	-8.1	19,019	-6.6	18,853	-0.9	19,948	+5.8	20,227	+1.4	20,782	+2.7
Total estimated part-time faculty	6,478	-5.4	6,077	-6.2	6,975	+14.8	8,222	+17.9	10,608	+29.0	11,411	+7.6
Est. unfilled budgeted positions	689	-8.4	869	+26.1	789	-9.2	860	+9.0	986	+14.7	1,016	+3.0
BACCALAUREATE AND HIGHER DEGREE PROGRAMS[4]												
Total Number of Programs	611	-2.2	637	+4.3	638	+0.2	635	-0.5	558	-12.1	665	+19.2
Total estimated nurse-faculty (full-time and FTEs)[5]	11,346	-8.1	11,455	+1.0	11,573	+1.0	12,039	+4.0	13,550	+12.6	14,239	+5.1
Total estimated full-time faculty	9,786	-9.8	10,045	+2.6	10,053	+0.1	10,377	+3.2	10,986	+5.9	11,212	+2.1
Total estimated part-time faculty	3,120	+4.5	2,819	-9.6	3,040	+7.8	3,326	+9.4	5,128	+54.2	6,055	+18.1
Est. unfilled budgeted positions	441	-2.2	519	+17.7	469	-9.6	537	+14.5	661	+23.1	586	-11.3
ASSOCIATE DEGREE PROGRAMS												
Total Number of Programs	787	+0.5	796	+1.1	812	+2.0	838	+3.2	857	+2.3	876	+2.2
Total estimated nurse-faculty (full-time and FTEs)[5]	8,516	+6.0	7,961	-6.5	8,713	+9.4	9,746	+11.9	10,372	+6.4	10,338	-0.3
Total estimated full-time faculty	7,153	+5.6	6,566	-8.2	6,957	+6.0	7,546	+8.5	7,849	+4.0	7,917	+0.9
Total estimated part-time faculty	2,725	+4.2	2,790	+2.4	3,511	+25.8	4,400	+25.3	5,046	+14.7	4,843	-4.0
Est. unfilled budgeted positions	156	-19.2	232	+48.7	229	-1.3	2626	14.4	303	15.6	368	+21.4
DIPLOMA PROGRAMS												
Total Number of Programs	256	-11.4	209	-18.4	157	-33.1	145	-7.6	129	-11.0	119	-7.7
Total estimated nurse-faculty (full-time and FTEs)[5]	3,639	-24.2	2,518	-30.8	2,179	-13.5	2,159	-0.9	2,071	-4.1	1,601	-22.7
Total estimated full-time faculty	3,342	-23.7	2-291	-31.4	1,954	-147	1,910	-2.2	1,779	-6.9	1,408	-20.8
Total estimated part-time faculty	594	-28.9	453	-23.7	449	-0.9	498	+10.9	583	+17.1	388	-33.4
Est. unfilled budgeted positions	83	-22.4	109	+31.3	979	-11.0	54	-44.3	56	+3.7	46	-17.9

[1] As of January of each year indicated. Estimates are based on an extension of the data to a 100% response rate to control for differences in response rate in each biennial surv
[2] Excludes American Samoa, Guam, Puerto Rico and the Virgin Islands.
[3] Directors of programs not included in table.
[4] Includes masters programs and RN baccalaureate programs.
[5] Full-time equivalent (FTEs) are calculated by assuming each part-time faculty member is equivalent to one-half of a full-time faculty member.

Table 4
MEAN NUMBER OF FULL-TIME AND PART-TIME NURSE FACULTY AND UNFILLED POSITIONS
BY TYPE OF PROGRAM, 1978-1996[1]

STATUS OF FACULTY	MEAN NUMBER OF FACULTY PER PROGRAM									
	1978	1980	1982	1984	1986	1988	1990	1992	1994	1996
ALL REPORTING PROGRAMS										
Full-time faculty	15.1	14.7	14.2	13.2	12.4	11.6	11.7	12.3	9.6	9.6
Part-time faculty	3.3	3.5	3.7	4.1	3.9	3.7	4.3	5.1	5.2	5.3
Unfilled positions	0.6	0.5	0.5	0.4	0.4	0.5	0.5	0.6	0.4	0.5
BACCALAUREATE AND HIGHER DEGREE PROGRAMS										
Full-time faculty	23.3	22.0	20.3	17.4	16.2	15.8	15.7	16.4	19.7	16.9
Part-time faculty	5.1	4.9	4.8	4.7	5.2	4.5	4.8	5.3	9.2	9.1
Unfilled positions	1.2	0.9	0.9	0.7	0.7	0.8	0.7	0.9	1.2	0.9
ASSOCIATE DEGREE PROGRAMS										
Full-time faculty	9.7	9.3	9.1	8.9	9.1	8.3	8.6	9.0	9.2	9.0
Part-time faculty	2.6	2.9	3.3	3.8	3.5	3.5	4.3	5.3	5.9	5.5
Unfilled positions	0.3	0.3	0.3	0.3	0.2	0.3	0.3	0.3	0.4	0.4
DIPLOMA PROGRAMS										
Full-time faculty	15.8	15.7	15.6	15.7	13.8	11.0	12.4	13.2	13.8	11.8
Part-time faculty	2.6	2.7	2.7	3.0	2.3	2.2	2.9	3.4	4.5	3.3
Unfilled positions	0.4	0.4	0.4	0.4	0.3	0.5	0.6	0.4	0.4	0.4
PN/VN PROGRAMS										
Full-time faculty	N/A	N/A	N/A	N/A	N/A	N/A	N/A	N/A	4.1	4.1
Part-time faculty	N/A	N/A	N/A	N/A	N/A	N/A	N/A	N/A	2.5	2.3
Unfilled positions	N/A	N/A	N/A	N/A	N/A	N/A	N/A	N/A	0.1	0.2

[1] Excludes American Samoa, Guam, Puerto Rico and the Virgin Islands.

Table 5
FULL-TIME AND PART-TIME NURSE FACULTY AND UNFILLED POSITIONS BY PROGRAM TYPE, MEAN, STANDARD DEVIATION AND RANGE, 1996[1]

CATEGORY	FULL-TIME FACULTY	PART-TIME FACULTY	UNFILLED POSITIONS
ALL REPORTING PROGRAMS			
Number of Reporting Programs	2,060	2,060	2,041
Mean Number of Faculty Positions	9.6	5.3	0.5
Standard Deviation	10.4	7.3	1.3
Minimum Number of Faculty Positions	0.0	0.0	0.0
Maximum Number of Faculty Positions	106	78	15
BACCALAUREATE AND HIGHER DEGREE PROGRAMS			
Number of Reporting Programs	564	564	563
Mean Number of Faculty Positions	16.9	9.1	0.9
Standard Deviation	15.4	10.2	1.7
Minimum Number of Faculty Positions	0.0	0.0	0.0
Maximum Number of Faculty Positions	106	78	15
ASSOCIATE DEGREE PROGRAMS			
Number of Reporting Programs	685	685	678
Mean Number of Faculty Positions	9.0	5.5	0.4
Standard Deviation	5.8	6.3	1.2
Minimum Number of Faculty Positions	0.0	0.0	0.0
Maximum Number of Faculty Positions	61	50	13
DIPLOMA PROGRAMS			
Number of Reporting Programs	93	93	93
Mean Number of Faculty Positions	11.8	3.3	0.4
Standard Deviation	4.6	4.5	1.6
Minimum Number of Faculty Positions	1.0	0.0	0.0
Maximum Number of Faculty Positions	28	24	14
PN/VN PROGRAMS			
Number of Reporting Programs	718	718	707
Mean Number of Faculty Positions	4.1	2.3	0.2
Standard Deviation	4.4	3.3	0.6
Minimum Number of Faculty Positions	0.0	0.0	0.0
Maximum Number of Faculty Positions	89	42	10

[1] Excludes American Samoa, Guam, Puerto Rico and the Virgin Islands.

Table 6
NUMBER OF FULL-TIME AND PART-TIME FACULTY
IN ALL NURSING PROGRAMS BY STATE AND REGION, 1996[1]

JURISDICTION	NUMBER OF PROGRAMS	TOTAL FACULTY	FULL-TIME FACULTY	PART-TIME FACULTY
United States	2,060	30,644	19,735	10,909
North Atlantic	434	7,172	4,184	2,988
Midwest	571	8,670	5,474	3,196
South	772	10,564	7,470	3,094
West	283	4,238	2,607	1,631
Alabama	37	555	339	216
Alaska	2	38	27	11
Arizona	20	296	187	109
Arkansas	40	330	239	91
California	123	1,953	1,134	819
Colorado	18	305	160	145
Connecticut	28	440	263	177
Delaware	10	188	113	75
District of Columbia	5	132	94	38
Florida	61	1,067	686	381
Georgia	54	690	468	222
Hawaii	7	159	93	66
Idaho	11	132	105	27
Illinois	92	1,234	775	459
Indiana	60	1,049	691	358
Iowa	44	464	295	169
Kansas	42	579	439	140
Kentucky	42	566	397	169
Louisiana	49	623	536	87
Maine	15	152	105	47
Maryland	28	603	374	229
Massachusetts	56	961	490	471
Michigan	59	1,364	653	711
Minnesota	38	458	307	151
Mississippi	28	446	398	48
Missouri	77	812	576	236
Montana	5	23	18	5
Nebraska	16	288	236	52
Nevada	7	109	74	35
New Hampshire	9	131	88	43
New Jersey	54	780	477	303
New Mexico	19	205	142	63
New York	122	2,253	1,165	1,088
North Carolina	73	841	545	296
North Dakota	11	163	119	44
Ohio	86	1,473	873	600
Oklahoma	43	372	256	116
Oregon	17	350	225	125
Pennsylvania	123	1,856	1,199	657
Rhode Island	5	216	150	66
South Carolina	36	430	305	125
South Dakota	12	201	112	89
Tennessee	47	705	521	184
Texas	125	1,964	1,542	422
Utah	8	119	94	25
Vermont	7	63	40	23
Virginia	79	1,042	619	423
Washington	34	460	285	175
West Virginia	30	330	245	85
Wisconsin	34	585	398	187
Wyoming	12	89	63	26
American Samoa	1	15	3	12
Guam	0	0	0	0
Puerto Rico	20	219	151	68
Virgin Islands	3	24	11	13

[1] Territories omitted from total.

Table 7
NUMBER OF FULL-TIME AND PART-TIME FACULTY
IN BACCALAUREATE AND HIGHER DEGREE PROGRAMS BY STATE AND REGION, 1996[1]

JURISDICTION	NUMBER OF PROGRAMS	TOTAL FACULTY	FULL-TIME FACULTY	PART-TIME FACULTY
United States	564	14,644	9,509	5,135
North Atlantic	138	3,452	1,939	1,513
Midwest	176	4,222	2,832	1,390
South	189	4,858	3,435	1,423
West	61	2,112	1,303	809
Alabama	8	223	163	60
Alaska	1	30	21	9
Arizona	3	104	75	29
Arkansas	7	128	95	33
California	26	916	514	402
Colorado	5	171	120	51
Connecticut	11	299	162	137
Delaware	3	90	43	47
District of Columbia	3	118	83	35
Florida	13	385	262	123
Georgia	16	355	257	98
Hawaii	2	121	61	60
Idaho	4	72	54	18
Illinois	29	540	332	208
Indiana	23	570	380	190
Iowa	15	206	144	62
Kansas	13	311	240	71
Kentucky	11	257	165	92
Louisiana	13	332	263	69
Maine	6	89	61	28
Maryland	9	325	216	109
Massachusetts	16	425	207	218
Michigan	16	605	341	264
Minnesota	9	215	147	68
Mississippi	8	178	142	36
Missouri	22	391	294	97
Montana	0	0	0	0
Nebraska	5	205	173	32
Nevada	3	63	47	16
New Hampshire	4	65	43	22
New Jersey	18	286	171	115
New Mexico	3	84	54	30
New York	40	1,122	555	567
North Carolina	13	336	235	101
North Dakota	7	134	104	30
Ohio	18	545	377	168
Oklahoma	10	158	117	41
Oregon	4	251	157	94
Pennsylvania	32	783	507	276
Rhode Island	3	148	84	64
South Carolina	10	223	170	53
South Dakota	5	127	68	59
Tennessee	18	453	334	119
Texas	26	800	596	204
Utah	2	59	48	11
Vermont	2	27	23	4
Virginia	17	509	282	227
Washington	7	222	136	86
West Virginia	10	196	138	58
Wisconsin	14	373	232	141
Wyoming	1	19	16	3
American Samoa	0	0	0	0
Guam	0	0	0	0
Puerto Rico	8	141	97	44
Virgin Islands	0	0	0	0

[1] Territories omitted from total.

Table 8
NUMBER OF FULL-TIME AND PART-TIME FACULTY
IN ASSOCIATE DEGREE PROGRAMS BY STATE AND REGION, 1996[1]

JURISDICTION	NUMBER OF PROGRAMS	TOTAL FACULTY	FULL-TIME FACULTY	PART-TIME FACULTY
United States	685	9,978	6,191	3,787
North Atlantic	120	2,070	1,188	882
Midwest	193	2,836	1,624	1,212
South	249	3,628	2,479	1,149
West	123	1,444	900	544
Alabama	15	171	94	77
Alaska	1	8	6	2
Arizona	8	105	55	50
Arkansas	11	119	89	30
California	55	737	457	280
Colorado	5	66	17	49
Connecticut	5	73	42	31
Delaware	4	61	42	19
District of Columbia	0	0	0	0
Florida	22	476	274	202
Georgia	16	227	135	92
Hawaii	3	30	26	4
Idaho	4	47	41	6
Illinois	31	408	275	133
Indiana	22	349	222	127
Iowa	12	133	70	63
Kansas	16	176	130	46
Kentucky	19	245	180	65
Louisiana	9	172	158	14
Maine	6	50	35	15
Maryland	11	215	117	98
Massachusetts	19	354	176	178
Michigan	26	508	199	309
Minnesota	12	141	100	41
Mississippi	14	230	221	9
Missouri	21	229	144	85
Montana	1	8	7	1
Nebraska	5	46	34	12
Nevada	4	46	27	19
New Hampshire	4	58	41	17
New Jersey	12	238	132	106
New Mexico	11	90	62	28
New York	46	773	431	342
North Carolina	35	381	225	156
North Dakota	0	0	0	0
Ohio	29	604	276	328
Oklahoma	14	135	85	50
Oregon	8	70	46	24
Pennsylvania	21	396	231	165
Rhode Island	1	52	52	0
South Carolina	11	142	92	50
South Dakota	5	65	38	27
Tennessee	10	160	112	48
Texas	41	629	506	123
Utah	2	37	31	6
Vermont	2	15	6	9
Virginia	13	235	119	116
Washington	14	153	90	63
West Virginia	8	91	72	19
Wisconsin	14	177	136	41
Wyoming	7	47	35	12
American Samoa	0	0	0	0
Guam	0	0	0	0
Puerto Rico	5	51	37	14
Virgin Islands	1	7	5	2

[1] Territories omitted from total.

Table 9
NUMBER OF FULL-TIME AND PART-TIME FACULTY
IN DIPLOMA PROGRAMS BY STATE AND REGION, 1996[1]

JURISDICTION	NUMBER OF PROGRAMS	TOTAL FACULTY	FULL-TIME FACULTY	PART-TIME FACULTY
United States	93	1,403	1,100	303
North Atlantic	52	775	577	198
Midwest	22	334	276	58
South	18	276	229	47
West	1	18	18	0
Alabama	0	0	0	0
Alaska	0	0	0	0
Arizona	0	0	0	0
Arkansas	1	11	10	1
California	1	18	18	0
Colorado	0	0	0	0
Connecticut	2	25	17	8
Delaware	1	10	10	0
District of Columbia	0	0	0	0
Florida	0	0	0	0
Georgia	0	0	0	0
Hawaii	0	0	0	0
Idaho	0	0	0	0
Illinois	4	53	46	7
Indiana	1	22	21	1
Iowa	4	48	34	14
Kansas	0	0	0	0
Kentucky	0	0	0	0
Louisiana	1	11	11	0
Maine	0	0	0	0
Maryland	1	7	6	1
Massachusetts	6	101	60	41
Michigan	1	15	11	4
Minnesota	0	0	0	0
Mississippi	0	0	0	0
Missouri	3	48	40	8
Montana	0	0	0	0
Nebraska	0	0	0	0
Nevada	0	0	0	0
New Hampshire	0	0	0	0
New Jersey	12	194	130	64
New Mexico	0	0	0	0
New York	5	57	44	13
North Carolina	3	51	35	16
North Dakota	0	0	0	0
Ohio	9	148	124	24
Oklahoma	0	0	0	0
Oregon	0	0	0	0
Pennsylvania	25	372	302	70
Rhode Island	1	16	14	2
South Carolina	0	0	0	0
South Dakota	0	0	0	0
Tennessee	2	22	18	4
Texas	2	54	48	6
Utah	0	0	0	0
Vermont	0	0	0	0
Virginia	8	120	101	19
Washington	0	0	0	0
West Virginia	0	0	0	0
Wisconsin	0	0	0	0
Wyoming	0	0	0	0
American Samoa	0	0	0	0
Guam	0	0	0	0
Puerto Rico	0	0	0	0
Virgin Islands	0	0	0	0

[1] Territories omitted from total.

35

Table 10

NUMBER OF FULL-TIME AND PART-TIME FACULTY IN PN/VN NURSING PROGRAMS BY STATE AND REGION, 1996[1]

JURISDICTION	NUMBER OF PROGRAMS	TOTAL FACULTY	FULL-TIME FACULTY	PART-TIME FACULTY
United States	718	4,619	2,935	1,684
North Atlantic	124	875	480	395
Midwest	180	1,278	742	536
South	316	1,802	1,327	475
West	98	664	386	278
Alabama	14	161	82	79
Alaska	0	0	0	0
Arizona	9	87	57	30
Arkansas	21	72	45	27
California	41	282	145	137
Colorado	8	68	23	45
Connecticut	10	43	42	1
Delaware	2	27	18	9
District of Columbia	2	14	11	3
Florida	26	206	150	56
Georgia	22	108	76	32
Hawaii	2	8	6	2
Idaho	3	13	10	3
Illinois	28	233	122	111
Indiana	14	108	68	40
Iowa	13	77	47	30
Kansas	13	92	69	23
Kentucky	12	64	52	12
Louisiana	26	108	104	4
Maine	3	13	9	4
Maryland	7	56	35	21
Massachusetts	15	81	47	34
Michigan	16	236	102	134
Minnesota	17	102	60	42
Mississippi	6	38	35	3
Missouri	31	144	98	46
Montana	4	15	11	4
Nebraska	6	37	29	8
Nevada	0	0	0	0
New Hampshire	1	8	4	4
New Jersey	12	62	44	18
New Mexico	5	31	26	5
New York	31	301	135	166
North Carolina	22	73	50	23
North Dakota	4	29	15	14
Ohio	30	176	96	80
Oklahoma	19	79	54	25
Oregon	5	29	22	7
Pennsylvania	45	305	159	146
Rhode Island	0	0	0	0
South Carolina	15	65	43	22
South Dakota	2	9	6	3
Tennessee	17	70	57	13
Texas	56	481	392	89
Utah	4	23	15	8
Vermont	3	21	11	10
Virginia	41	178	117	61
Washington	13	85	59	26
West Virginia	12	43	35	8
Wisconsin	6	35	30	5
Wyoming	4	23	12	11
American Samoa	1	15	3	12
Guam	0	0	0	0
Puerto Rico	7	27	17	10
Virgin Islands	2	17	6	11

36

[1] Territories omitted from total.

Table 11

UNFILLED NURSE FACULTY BUDGETED POSITIONS PER 100 FULL-TIME FACULTY BY REGION, 1986-1996[1,2]

REGION BY YEAR	TOTAL FULL-TIME FACULTY REPORTED	TOTAL BUDGETED VACANCIES REPORTED	VACANCIES PER 100 FULL-TIME FACULTY
All Regions			
1986	18,374	611	3.3
1988	16,821	768	4.6
1990	16,723	700	4.2
1992	16,836	726	4.1
1994	20,205	920	4.4
1996	19,735	994	4.8
North Atlantic			
1986	5,146	96	1.9
1988	4,083	132	3.2
1990	4,185	132	3.2
1992	3,704	142	3.7
1994	4,314	175	3.9
1996	4,184	175	4.0
Midwest			
1986	5,072	182	3.6
1988	4,638	212	4.6
1990	4,660	190	4.1
1992	4,746	177	3.6
1994	5,577	249	4.3
1996	5,474	219	3.8
South			
1986	5,731	235	4.1
1988	5,606	313	5.6
1990	5,626	291	5.2
1992	5,895	317	5.1
1994	7,629	348	4.4
1996	7,470	442	5.6
West			
1986	2,425	98	4.0
1988	2,494	111	4.5
1990	2,245	87	3.9
1992	2,491	90	3.5
1994	2,685	148	5.2
1996	2,607	158	5.7

[1] Excludes American Samoa, Guam, Puerto Rico and the Virgin Islands
[2] Vacancy rates were calculated as follows: Budgeted Vacancies/total Full-Time Positions + Budgeted Vacancies.

Table 12
UNFILLED NURSE FACULTY POSITIONS PER 100 FULL-TIME FACULTY BY PROGRAM TYPE, 1996[1,2]

NUMBER OF BUDGETED POSITIONS	NUMBER OF FACULTY	NUMBER OF BUDGETED VACANCIES	VACANCIES PER 100 FACULTY
ALL REPORTING PROGRAMS			
20,729	19,735	994	4.8
BACCALAUREATE AND HIGHER DEGREE PROGRAMS			
10,006	9,509	497	5.0
ASSOCIATE DEGREE PROGRAMS			
6,479	6,191	288	4.4
DIPLOMA PROGRAMS			
1,136	1,100	36	3.2
PN/VN PROGRAMS			
3,108	2,935	173	5.6

[1] Excludes American Samoa, Guam, Puerto Rico and the Virgin Islands.
[2] Vacancy rates were calculated as follows:
Budgeted Vacancies/Total Full-Time Positions + Budgeted Vacancies.

38

Table 13A
PRIMARY TEACHING RESPONSIBILITIES OF ALL NURSING FACULTY
ACCORDING TO HIGHEST EARNED CREDENTIAL, 1996[1]

FACULTY CREDENTIALS	ALL FACULTY REPORTED		PRIMARY TEACHING RESPONSIBILITY									
			PRACTICAL NURSING		DIPLOMA		ASSOCIATE DEGREE		BACCALAUREATE		GRADUATE	
	NUMBER	PERCENT	NUMBER	PERCENT	NUMBER	PERCENT	NUMBER	PERCENT	NUMBER	PERCENT	NUMBER	PERCENT
All Credentials	26,278	100.0	3,813	14.5	1,287	4.9	8,893	33.8	9,198	35.0	3,087	11.7
Doctorate	5,370	100.0	47	0.9	43	0.8	472	8.8	2,621	48.8	2,187	40.7
Masters	16,261	100.0	1,268	7.8	1,104	6.8	6,764	41.6	6,258	38.5	867	5.3
Baccalaureate	3,866	100.0	1,841	47.6	126	3.3	1,572	40.7	304	7.9	23	0.6
Other Credential	781	100.0	657	84.1	14	1.8	85	10.9	15	1.9	10	1.3

[1] Excludes American Samoa, Guam, Puerto Rico and the Virgin Islands.

Table 13B
PRIMARY TEACHING RESPONSIBILITIES OF FULL-TIME NURSING FACULTY
ACCORDING TO HIGHEST EARNED CREDENTIAL, 1996[1]

FACULTY CREDENTIALS	FULL-TIME FACULTY REPORTED		PRIMARY TEACHING RESPONSIBILITY									
			PRACTICAL NURSING		DIPLOMA		ASSOCIATE DEGREE		BACCALAUREATE		GRADUATE	
	NUMBER	PERCENT	NUMBER	PERCENT	NUMBER	PERCENT	NUMBER	PERCENT	NUMBER	PERCENT	NUMBER	PERCENT
All Credentials	18,760	100.0	2,694	14.4	1,046	5.6	6,127	32.7	6,452	34.4	2,441	13.0
Doctorate	4,840	100.0	39	0.8	37	0.8	411	8.5	2,382	49.2	1,971	40.7
Masters	11,666	100.0	1,041	8.9	915	7.8	5,243	44.9	4,008	34.4	459	3.9
Baccalaureate	1,768	100.0	1,169	66.1	84	4.8	449	25.4	59	3.3	7	0.4
Other Credential	486	100.0	445	91.6	10	2.1	24	4.9	3	0.6	4	0.8

[1] Excludes American Samoa, Guam, Puerto Rico and the Virgin Islands.

Table 13C
PRIMARY TEACHING RESPONSIBILITIES OF PART-TIME NURSING FACULTY
ACCORDING TO HIGHEST EARNED CREDENTIAL, 1996[1]

FACULTY CREDENTIALS	PART-TIME FACULTY REPORTED		PRIMARY TEACHING RESPONSIBILITY									
			PRACTICAL NURSING		DIPLOMA		ASSOCIATE DEGREE		BACCALAUREATE		GRADUATE	
	NUMBER	PERCENT	NUMBER	PERCENT	NUMBER	PERCENT	NUMBER	PERCENT	NUMBER	PERCENT	NUMBER	PERCENT
All Credentials	7,463	100.0	1,117	15.0	238	3.2	2,737	36.7	2,730	36.6	641	8.6
Doctorate	520	100.0	8	1.5	6	1.2	59	11.3	235	45.2	212	40.8
Masters	4,557	100.0	227	5.0	186	4.1	1,495	32.8	2,242	49.2	407	8.9
Baccalaureate	2,091	100.0	670	32.0	42	2.0	1,122	53.7	241	11.5	16	0.8
Other Credential	295	100.0	212	71.9	4	1.4	61	20.7	12	4.1	6	2.0

[1] Excludes American Samoa, Guam, Puerto Rico and the Virgin Islands.

Table 14
RACIAL/ETHNIC BACKGROUND OF ADMINISTRATORS
BY TYPE OF PROGRAM AND REGION, 1996[1]

NLN Region	Total United States		American Indian or Alaskan Native		Asian or Pacific Islander		Black Non-Hispanic)		Hispanic		White (Other Than Hispanic)	
	Number	Percent	Number	Percent	Number	Percent	Number	Percent	Number	Percent	Number	Percent
ALL REPORTING PROGRAMS												
All Regions	1,722	100.0	9	0.5	22	1.3	109	6.3	28	1.6	1,554	90.2
North Atlantic	366	100.0	0	0.0	2	0.5	17	4.6	5	1.4	342	93.4
Midwest	466	100.0	1	0.2	5	1.1	20	4.3	4	0.9	436	93.6
South	661	100.0	6	0.9	4	0.6	66	10.0	12	1.8	573	86.7
West	229	100.0	2	0.9	11	4.8	6	2.6	7	3.1	203	88.6
BACCALAUREATE AND HIGHER DEGREE PROGRAMS												
All Regions	551	100.0	1	0.2	7	1.3	32	5.8	6	1.1	505	91.7
North Atlantic	130	100.0	0	0.0	2	1.5	7	5.4	2	1.5	119	91.5
Midwest	171	100.0	0	0.0	1	0.6	6	3.5	0	0.0	164	95.9
South	189	100.0	1	0.5	1	0.5	19	10.1	4	2.1	164	86.8
West	61	100.0	0	0.0	3	4.9	0	0.0	0	0.0	58	95.1
ASSOCIATE DEGREE PROGRAMS												
All Regions	554	100.0	5	0.9	10	1.8	28	5.1	14	2.5	497	89.7
North Atlantic	97	100.0	0	0.0	0	0.0	3	3.1	2	2.1	92	94.8
Midwest	150	100.0	0	0.0	2	1.3	6	4.0	2	1.3	140	93.3
South	212	100.0	3	1.4	3	1.4	17	8.0	5	2.4	184	86.8
West	95	100.0	2	2.1	5	5.3	2	2.1	5	5.3	81	85.3
DIPLOMA PROGRAMS												
All Regions	75	100.0	0	0.0	0	0.0	1	1.3	1	1.3	73	97.3
North Atlantic	42	100.0	0	0.0	0	0.0	0	0.0	0	0.0	42	100.0
Midwest	17	100.0	0	0.0	0	0.0	0	0.0	1	5.9	16	94.1
South	15	100.0	0	0.0	0	0.0	1	6.7	0	0.0	14	93.3
West	1	100.0	0	0.0	0	0.0	0	0.0	0	0.0	1	100.0
PN\VN NURSING PROGRAMS												
All Regions	542	100.0	3	0.6	5	0.9	48	8.9	7	1.3	479	88.4
North Atlantic	97	100.0	0	0.0	0	0.0	7	7.2	1	1.0	89	91.8
Midwest	128	100.0	1	0.8	2	1.6	8	6.3	1	0.8	116	90.6
South	245	100.0	2	0.8	0	0.0	29	11.8	3	1.2	211	86.1
West	72	100.0	0	0.0	3	4.2	4	5.6	2	2.8	63	87.5

[1] Excludes American Samoa, Guam, Puerto Rico and the Virgin Islands

Table 15
RACIAL/ETHNIC BACKGROUND OF FULL-TIME FACULTY
BY TYPE OF PROGRAM AND REGION, 1996[1]

NLN REGION	Total Full-Time Faculty Reported		American Indian or Alaskan Native		Asian/Pacific Islander		Black (Non-Hispanic)		Hispanic		White, Other than Hispanic	
	Number	Percent	Number	Percent	Number	Percent	Number	Percent	Number	Percent	Number	Percent
ALL REPORTING PROGRAMS												
All Regions	17,493	100.0	66	0.4	250	1.4	1,051	6.0	227	1.3	15,899	90.9
North Atlantic	3,735	100.0	6	0.2	39	1.0	158	4.2	26	0.7	3,506	93.9
Midwest	4,980	100.0	15	0.3	53	1.1	186	3.7	28	0.6	4,698	94.3
South	6,642	100.0	28	0.4	55	0.8	613	9.2	114	1.7	5,832	87.8
West	2,136	100.0	17	0.8	103	4.8	94	4.4	59	2.8	1,863	87.2
BACCALAUREATE AND HIGHER DEGREE PROGRAMS												
All Regions	8,609	100.0	26	0.3	122	1.4	434	5.0	79	0.9	7,948	92.3
North Atlantic	1,810	100.0	2	0.1	17	0.9	87	4.8	13	0.7	1,691	93.4
Midwest	2,669	100.0	8	0.3	30	1.1	92	3.4	8	0.3	2,531	94.8
South	3,090	100.0	9	0.3	30	1.0	229	7.4	40	1.3	2,782	90.0
West	1,040	100.0	7	0.7	45	4.3	26	2.5	18	1.7	944	90.8
ASSOCIATE DEGREE PROGRAMS												
All Regions	5,463	100.0	26	0.5	82	1.5	341	6.2	80	1.5	4,934	90.3
North Atlantic	1,024	100.0	3	0.3	11	1.1	42	4.1	3	0.3	965	94.2
Midwest	1,456	100.0	5	0.3	18	1.2	56	3.8	9	0.6	1,368	94.0
South	2,228	100.0	11	0.5	14	0.6	201	9.0	41	1.8	1,961	88.0
West	755	100.0	7	0.9	39	5.2	42	5.6	27	3.6	640	84.8
DIPLOMA PROGRAMS												
All Regions	998	100.0	2	0.2	20	2.0	37	3.7	24	2.4	915	91.7
North Atlantic	500	100.0	0	0.0	8	1.6	12	2.4	7	1.4	473	94.6
Midwest	257	100.0	0	0.0	3	1.2	4	1.6	10	3.9	240	93.4
South	223	100.0	1	0.4	5	2.2	17	7.6	4	1.8	196	87.9
West	18	100.0	1	5.6	4	22.2	4	22.2	3	16.7	6	33.3
PN/VN PROGRAMS												
All Regions	2,423	100.0	12	0.5	26	1.1	239	9.9	44	1.8	2,102	86.8
North Atlantic	401	100.0	1	0.2	3	0.7	17	4.2	3	0.7	377	94.0
Midwest	598	100.0	2	0.3	2	0.3	34	5.7	1	0.2	559	93.5
South	1,101	100.0	7	0.6	6	0.5	166	15.1	29	2.6	893	81.1
West	323	100.0	2	0.6	15	4.6	22	6.8	11	3.4	273	84.5

[1] Excludes American Samoa, Guam, Puerto Rico and the Virgin Islands

Table 16
RACIAL/ETHNIC BACKGROUND OF PART-TIME FACULTY BY TYPE OF PROGRAM AND REGION, 1996[1]

NLN REGION	Total Part-Time Faculty Reported		American Indian or Alaskan Native		Asian/Pacific Islander		Black (Non-Hispanic)		Hispanic		White, Other than Hispanic	
	Number	Percent	Number	Percent	Number	Percent	Number	Percent	Number	Percent	Number	Percent
ALL REPORTING PROGRAMS												
All Regions	7,572	100.0	28	0.4	151	2.0	357	4.7	122	1.6	6,914	91.3
North Atlantic	1,909	100.0	2	0.1	21	1.1	79	4.1	17	0.9	1,790	93.8
Midwest	2,390	100.0	5	0.2	29	1.2	70	2.9	10	0.4	2,276	95.2
South	2,121	100.0	14	0.7	41	1.9	158	7.4	49	2.3	1,859	87.6
West	1,152	100.0	7	0.6	60	5.2	50	4.3	46	4.0	989	85.9
BACCALAUREATE AND HIGHER DEGREE PROGRAMS												
All Regions	3,571	100.0	8	0.2	68	1.9	129	3.6	53	1.5	3,313	92.8
North Atlantic	865	100.0	2	0.2	10	1.2	32	3.7	12	1.4	809	93.5
Midwest	1,125	100.0	4	0.4	12	1.1	28	2.5	4	0.4	1,077	95.7
South	1,013	100.0	1	0.1	16	1.6	54	5.3	14	1.4	928	91.6
West	568	100.0	1	0.2	30	5.3	15	2.6	23	4.0	499	87.9
ASSOCIATE DEGREE PROGRAMS												
All Regions	2,584	100.0	13	0.5	59	2.3	120	4.6	37	1.4	2,355	91.1
North Atlantic	596	100.0	0	0.0	7	1.2	20	3.4	2	0.3	567	95.1
Midwest	859	100.0	0	0.0	14	1.6	29	3.4	1	0.1	815	94.9
South	750	100.0	11	1.5	20	2.7	50	6.7	21	2.8	648	86.4
West	379	100.0	2	0.5	18	4.7	21	5.5	13	3.4	325	85.8
DIPLOMA PROGRAMS												
All Regions	230	100	0	0.0	4	1.7	4	1.7	6	2.6	216	93.9
North Atlantic	132	100	0	0.0	2	1.5	1	0.8	1	0.8	128	97.0
Midwest	55	100	0	0.0	1	1.8	2	3.6	5	9.1	47	85.5
South	43	100	0	0.0	1	2.3	1	2.3	0	0.0	41	95.3
West	0	0.0	0	0.0	0	0.0	0	0.0	0	0.0	0	0.0
PN/VN PROGRAMS												
All Regions	1,187	100.0	7	0.6	20	1.7	104	8.8	26	2.2	1,030	86.8
North Atlantic	316	100.0	0	0.0	2	0.6	26	8.2	2	0.6	286	90.5
Midwest	351	100.0	1	0.3	2	0.6	11	3.1	0	0.0	337	96.0
South	315	100.0	2	0.6	4	1.3	53	16.8	14	4.4	242	76.8
West	205	100.0	4	2.0	12	5.9	14	6.8	10	4.9	165	80.5

[1] Excludes American Samoa, Guam, Puerto Rico and the Virgin Islands

Table 17
FULL-TIME FACULTY BY GENDER, TYPE OF PROGRAM AND REGION, 1996[1]

NLN REGION	NUMBER OF RESPONDING PROGRAMS	TOTAL NUMBER OF FULL-TIME FACULTY		MALE		FEMALE	
		Number	Percent	Number	Percent	Number	Percent
ALL REPORTING PROGRAMS							
All Regions	2,016	17,561	100.0	561	3.2	17,000	96.8
North Atlantic	424	3,767	100.0	95	2.5	3,672	97.5
Midwest	558	4,993	100.0	101	2.0	4,892	98.0
South	757	6,648	100.0	258	3.9	6,390	96.1
West	277	2,153	100.0	107	5.0	2,046	95.0
BACCALAUREATE AND HIGHER DEGREE PROGRAMS							
All Regions	549	8,612	100.0	309	3.6	8,303	96.4
North Atlantic	134	1,814	100.0	63	3.5	1,751	96.5
Midwest	168	2,669	100.0	65	2.4	2,604	97.6
South	186	3,085	100.0	137	4.4	2,948	95.6
West	61	1,044	100.0	44	4.2	1,000	95.8
ASSOCIATE DEGREE PROGRAMS							
All Regions	677	5,525	100.0	128	2.3	5,397	97.7
North Atlantic	120	1,051	100.0	13	1.2	1,038	98.8
Midwest	190	1,470	100.0	21	1.4	1,449	98.6
South	246	2,236	100.0	47	2.1	2,189	97.9
West	121	768	100.0	47	6.1	721	93.9
DIPLOMA PROGRAMS							
All Regions	92	997	100.0	27	2.7	970	97.3
North Atlantic	52	500	100.0	15	3.0	485	97.0
Midwest	22	256	100.0	6	2.3	250	97.7
South	17	223	100.0	5	2.2	218	97.8
West	1	18	100.0	1	5.6	17	94.4
PN/VN PROGRAMS							
All Regions	698	2,427	100.0	97	4.0	2,330	96.0
North Atlantic	118	402	100.0	4	1.0	398	99.0
Midwest	178	598	100.0	9	1.5	589	98.5
South	308	1,104	100.0	69	6.3	1,035	93.8
West	94	323	100.0	15	4.6	308	95.4

[1] Excludes American Samoa, Guam, Puerto Rico and the Virgin Islands

Table 18
PART-TIME FACULTY BY GENDER, TYPE OF PROGRAM AND REGION, 1996[1]

NLN REGION	NUMBER OF RESPONDING PROGRAMS	TOTAL NUMBER OF FULL-TIME FACULTY		MALE		FEMALE	
		Number	Percent	Number	Percent	Number	Percent
ALL REPORTING PROGRAMS							
All Regions	1,571	7,625	100.0	347	4.6	7,278	95.4
North Atlantic	338	1,928	100.0	88	4.6	1,840	95.4
Midwest	455	2,410	100.0	89	3.7	2,321	96.3
South	552	2,124	100.0	111	5.2	2,013	94.8
West	226	1,163	100.0	59	5.1	1,104	94.9
BACCALAUREATE AND HIGHER DEGREE PROGRAMS							
All Regions	469	3,601	100.0	196	5.4	3,405	94.6
North Atlantic	115	880	100.0	49	5.6	831	94.4
Midwest	143	1,132	100.0	45	4.0	1,087	96.0
South	154	1,016	100.0	65	6.4	951	93.6
West	57	573	100.0	37	6.5	536	93.5
ASSOCIATE DEGREE PROGRAMS							
All Regions	567	2,609	100.0	94	3.6	2,515	96.4
North Atlantic	102	600	100.0	19	3.2	581	96.8
Midwest	159	872	100.0	34	3.9	838	96.1
South	207	751	100.0	28	3.7	723	96.3
West	99	386	100.0	13	3.4	373	96.6
DIPLOMA PROGRAMS							
All Regions	63	230	100.0	8	3.5	222	96.5
North Atlantic	35	132	100.0	4	3.0	128	97.0
Midwest	15	55	100.0	1	1.8	54	98.2
South	13	43	100.0	3	7.0	40	93.0
West	0	0	0.0	0	0.0	0	0.0
PN/VN PROGRAMS							
All Regions	472	1,185	100.0	49	4.1	1.136	95.9
North Atlantic	86	316	100.0	16	5.1	300	94.9
Midwest	138	351	100.0	9	2.6	342	97.4
South	178	314	100.0	15	4.8	299	95.2
West	70	204	100.0	9	4.4	195	95.6

[1] Excludes American Samoa, Guam, Puerto Rico and the Virgin Islands

Table 19
NUMBER AND PERCENT OF FULL-TIME NURSE AND NON-NURSE FACULTY BY TYPE OF PROGRAM AND REGION, 1996[1]

NLN REGION	TOTAL FULL-TIME FACULTY		NURSE FACULTY		NON-NURSE FACULTY		TOTAL PART-TIME FACULTY		NURSE FACULTY		NON-NURSE FACULTY	
	Number	Percent	Number	Percent	Number	Percent	Number	Percent	Number	Percent	Number	Percent
ALL REPORTING PROGRAMS												
All Regions	19,735	100.0	19,323	97.9	412	2.1	10,909	100.0	10,320	94.6	589	5.4
North Atlantic	4,184	100.0	4,074	97.4	110	2.6	2,988	100.0	2,809	94.0	179	6.0
Midwest	5,474	100.0	5,357	97.9	117	2.1	3,196	100.0	3,052	95.5	144	4.5
South	7,470	100.0	7,344	98.3	126	1.7	3,094	100.0	2,917	94.3	177	5.7
West	2,607	100.0	2,548	97.7	59	2.3	1,631	100.0	1,542	94.5	89	5.5
BACCALAUREATE AND HIGHER DEGREE PROGRAMS												
All Regions	9,509	100.0	9,352	98.3	157	1.7	5,135	100.0	4,799	93.5	336	6.5
North Atlantic	1,939	100.0	1,910	98.5	29	1.5	1,513	100.0	1,417	93.7	96	6.3
Midwest	2,832	100.0	2,806	99.1	26	0.9	1,390	100.0	1,323	95.2	67	4.8
South	3,435	100.0	3,376	98.3	59	1.7	1,423	100.0	1,309	92.0	114	8.0
West	1,303	100.0	1,260	96.7	43	3.3	809	100.0	750	92.7	59	7.3
ASSOCIATE DEGREE PROGRAMS												
All Regions	6,191	100.0	6,108	98.7	83	1.3	3,787	100.0	3,693	97.5	94	2.5
North Atlantic	1,188	100.0	1,162	97.8	26	2.2	882	100.0	857	97.2	25	2.8
Midwest	1,624	100.0	1,599	98.5	25	1.5	1,212	100.0	1,171	96.6	41	3.4
South	2,479	100.0	2,460	99.2	19	0.8	1,149	100.0	1,131	98.4	18	1.6
West	900	100.0	887	98.6	13	1.4	544	100.0	534	98.2	10	1.8
DIPLOMA PROGRAMS												
All Regions	1,100	100.0	1,027	93.4	73	6.6	303	100.0	267	88.1	36	11.9
North Atlantic	577	100.0	541	93.8	36	6.2	198	100.0	169	85.4	29	14.6
Midwest	276	100.0	246	89.1	30	10.9	58	100.0	56	96.6	2	3.4
South	229	100.0	222	96.9	7	3.1	47	100.0	42	89.4	5	10.6
West	18	100.0	18	100.0	0	0.0	0	0	0	0.0	0	0.0
PN/VN NURSING PROGRAMS												
All Regions	2,935	100.0	2,836	96.6	99	3.4	1,684	100.0	1,561	92.7	123	7.3
North Atlantic	480	100.0	461	96.0	19	4.0	395	100.0	366	92.7	29	7.3
Midwest	742	100.0	706	95.1	36	4.9	536	100.0	502	93.7	34	6.3
South	1,327	100.0	1,286	96.9	41	3.1	475	100.0	435	91.6	40	8.4
West	386	100.0	383	99.2	3	0.8	278	100.0	258	92.8	20	7.2

[1] Excludes American Samoa, Guam, Puerto Rico and the Virgin Islands

45

Table 20

HIGHEST EARNED CREDENTIAL OF NURSING EDUCATION ADMINISTRATORS BY TYPE OF PROGRAM, 1978-1996[1]

YEAR	TOTAL ADMINISTRATORS REPORTED		HIGHEST EARNED CREDENTIAL					
			DOCTORATE		MASTER'S		OTHER	
	Number	Percent	Number	Percent	Number	Percent	Number	Percent
ALL REPORTING PROGRAMS								
1978	1,270	100.0	297	23.4	939	73.9	34	2.7
1980	1,344	100.0	355	26.4	960	71.4	29	2.2
1982	1,348	100.0	432	32.1	898	66.6	18	1.3
1984	1,499	100.0	524	35.0	937	62.5	38	2.5
1986	1,439	100.0	601	41.8	821	57.1	17	0.1
1988	1,370	100.0	589	43.0	767	56.0	14	1.0
1990	1,365	100.0	603	44.2	743	54.4	19	1.4
1992	1,331	100.0	637	47.9	689	51.8	5	0.4
1994	2,040	100.0	644	31.6	1,135	55.6	261	12.8
1996	1,726	100.0	709	41.1	861	49.9	156	9.0
BACCALAUREATE AND HIGHER DEGREE PROGRAMS								
1978	343	100.0	239	69.7	102	29.7	2	0.6
1980	414	100.0	269	65.0	144	34.8	1	0.2
1982	453	100.0	321	70.9	132	29.1	0	0.0
1984	535	100.0	381	71.2	154	28.8	0	0.0
1986	547	100.0	423	77.3	122	22.3	2	0.4
1988	540	100.0	422	78.1	114	21.1	4	0.7
1990	523	100.0	453	86.6	65	12.4	5	1.0
1992	531	100.0	469	88.3	61	11.5	1	0.2
1994	421	100.0	387	91.9	31	7.4	3	0.7
1996	546	100.0	504	92.3	40	7.3	2	0.4
ASSOCIATE DEGREE PROGRAMS								
1978	590	100.0	50	8.5	526	89.1	14	2.4
1980	634	100.0	77	12.2	539	85.0	18	2.8
1982	620	100.0	99	16.0	511	82.4	10	1.6
1984	712	100.0	128	18.0	552	77.5	32	4.5
1986	678	100.0	154	22.7	514	75.8	10	1.3
1988	661	100.0	147	22.2	504	76.2	10	1.5
1990	694	100.0	129	18.6	553	79.7	12	1.7
1992	678	100.0	149	22.0	525	77.4	4	0.6
1994	726	100.0	183	25.2	537	74.0	6	0.8
1996	557	100.0	149	26.8	400	71.8	8	1.4
DIPLOMA PROGRAMS								
1978	337	100.0	8	2.4	311	92.3	18	5.3
1980	296	100.0	9	3.0	277	93.6	10	3.4
1982	275	100.0	12	4.4	255	92.7	8	2.9
1984	252	100.0	15	6.0	231	91.7	6	2.4
1986	214	100.0	24	11.2	185	86.4	5	2.3
1988	169	100.0	20	11.8	149	88.2	0	0.0
1990	148	100.0	21	14.2	125	84.5	2	1.3
1992	122	100.0	19	15.6	103	84.4	0	0.0
1994	112	100.0	20	17.9	91	81.3	1	0.9
1996	77	100.0	18	23.4	59	76.6	0	0.0
PN/VN								
1978	N/A	N/A	N/A	N/A	N/A	N/A	N/A	N/A
1980	N/A	N/A	N/A	N/A	N/A	N/A	N/A	N/A
1982	N/A	N/A	N/A	N/A	N/A	N/A	N/A	N/A
1984	N/A	N/A	N/A	N/A	N/A	N/A	N/A	N/A
1986	N/A	N/A	N/A	N/A	N/A	N/A	N/A	N/A
1988	N/A	N/A	N/A	N/A	N/A	N/A	N/A	N/A
1990	N/A	N/A	N/A	N/A	N/A	N/A	N/A	N/A
1992	N/A	N/A	N/A	N/A	N/A	N/A	N/A	N/A
1994	781	100.0	54	6.9	476	60.9	251	32.1
1996	546	100.0	38	7.0	362	66.3	146	26.7

[1] Excludes American Samoa, Guam, Puerto Rico and the Virgin Islands.

Table 21
HIGHEST EARNED CREDENTIAL OF FULL-TIME NURSE FACULTY BY TYPE OF PROGRAM, 1978-1996[1,2]

YEAR	TOTAL FACULTY REPORTED		HIGHEST EARNED CREDENTIAL							
			DOCTORATE		MASTER'S		BACCALAUREATE		OTHER	
	Number	Percent	Number	Percent	Number	Percent	Number	Percent	Number	Percent
ALL REPORTING PROGRAMS										
1978	20,217	100.0	1,062	5.3	12,637	62.5	5,865	29.0	653	3.2
1980	20,355	100.0	1,418	7.0	13,826	67.9	4,687	23.0	424	2.1
1982	19,742	100.0	1,657	8.4	14,085	71.3	3,751	19.0	249	1.3
1984	20,221	100.0	2,143	10.6	14,797	73.2	3,104	15.4	177	0.9
1986	17,978	100.0	2,404	13.0	13,480	75.0	1,969	10.7	125	0.6
1988	17,083	100.0	3,160	18.5	12,605	73.8	1,254	7.3	64	0.4
1990	16,656	100.0	3,565	21.4	11,890	71.4	1,247	6.9	54	0.3
1992	16,549	100.0	3,867	23.4	11,533	69.7	1,108	6.7	41	0.2
1994	19,961	100.0	4,222	21.2	12,607	63.2	2,562	12.8	570	2.9
1996	17,505	100.0	4,311	24.7	11,029	63.0	1,682	9.6	463	2.6
BACCALAUREATE AND HIGHER DEGREE PROGRAMS										
1978	8,794	100.0	992	11.3	7,072	80.4	717	8.2	13	0.1
1980	9,531	100.0	1,278	13.4	7,763	81.4	485	5.1	5	0.1
1982	9,502	100.0	1,533	16.1	7,647	80.5	321	3.4	1	0.0
1984	9,827	100.0	1,967	20.0	7,594	77.3	259	2.6	6	0.1
1986	9,184	100.0	2,176	23.7	6,844	74.5	164	1.8	0	0.0
1988	9,074	100.0	2,921	32.2	6,045	66.6	103	1.1	5	0.1
1990	8,594	100.0	3,240	37.7	5,272	61.3	67	0.8	15	0.2
1992	8,806	100.0	3,596	40.8	5,109	58.0	94	1.1	7	0.1
1994	8,489	100.0	3,822	45.0	4,587	54.0	77	0.9	3	0.0
1996	8,615	100.0	3,969	46.1	4,571	53.1	71	0.8	4	0.0
ASSOCIATE DEGREE PROGRAMS										
1978	5,939	100.0	56	0.9	3,795	63.9	1,927	32.5	161	2.7
1980	6,036	100.0	128	2.1	4,216	69.8	1,593	26.4	99	1.7
1982	5,863	100.0	108	1.8	4,394	74.9	1,295	22.1	66	1.2
1984	6,452	100.0	162	2.5	4,977	77.1	1,238	19.2	75	1.2
1986	5,907	100.0	200	3.4	4,729	80.1	929	15.7	52	0.9
1988	5,986	100.0	218	3.6	5,017	83.8	712	11.9	39	0.7
1990	6,208	100.0	303	4.9	5,157	83.0	725	11.7	23	0.4
1992	6,143	100.0	245	4.0	5,176	84.3	697	11.3	25	0.4
1994	6,712	100.0	325	4.8	5,657	84.3	695	10.4	35	0.5
1996	5,489	100.0	314	5.7	4,676	85.2	474	8.6	25	0.5
DIPLOMA PROGRAMS										
1978	5,484	100.0	14	0.3	1,770	32.3	3,221	58.7	479	8.7
1980	4.788	100.0	12	0.2	1,847	38.6	2,609	54.5	320	6.7
1982	4,377	100.0	16	0.3	2.044	46.7	2,135	48.8	182	4.2
1984	3,942	100.0	14	0.4	2,226	56.5	1,606	40.7	96	2.5
1986	2,884	100.0	28	1.0	1,907	66.1	876	30.4	73	2.5
1988	2,023	100.0	21	1.0	1,543	76.3	439	21.7	20	1.0
1990	1,854	100.0	22	1.2	1,461	78.8	355	19.1	16	0.9
1992	1,600	100.0	26	1.6	1,248	78.0	317	19.8	9	0.6
1994	1,555	100.0	44	2.8	1,277	82.1	230	14.8	4	0.3
1996	997	100.0	21	2.1	889	89.2	82	8.2	5	0.5
PN/VN PROGRAMS										
1978	N/A	N/A	N/A	N/A	N/A	N/A	N/A	N/A	N/A	N/A
1980	N/A	N/A	N/A	N/A	N/A	N/A	N/A	N/A	N/A	N/A
1982	N/A	N/A	N/A	N/A	N/A	N/A	N/A	N/A	N/A	N/A
1984	N/A	N/A	N/A	N/A	N/A	N/A	N/A	N/A	N/A	N/A
1986	N/A	N/A	N/A	N/A	N/A	N/A	N/A	N/A	N/A	N/A
1988	N/A	N/A	N/A	N/A	N/A	N/A	N/A	N/A	N/A	N/A
1990	N/A	N/A	N/A	N/A	N/A	N/A	N/A	N/A	N/A	N/A
1992	N/A	N/A	N/A	N/A	N/A	N/A	N/A	N/A	N/A	N/A
1994	3,205	100.0	31	1.0	1,086	33.9	1,560	48.7	528	16.5
1996	2,404	100.0	27	1.1	893	37.1	1,055	43.9	429	17.8

[1] Chief administrator of programs not included in this table.
[2] Excludes American Samoa, Guam, Puerto Rico and the Virgin Islands.

Table 22
HIGHEST EARNED CREDENTIAL OF PART-TIME NURSE FACULTY BY TYPE OF PROGRAM, 1978-1996[1]

YEAR	TOTAL PART-TIME FACULTY REPORTED		HIGHEST EARNED CREDENTIAL							
			DOCTORATE		MASTER'S		BACCALAUREATE		OTHER	
	Number	Percent	Number	Percent	Number	Percent	Number	Percent	Number	Percent
ALL REPORTING PROGRAMS										
1978	4,457	100.0	131	2.9	1,975	44.3	2,043	45.9	308	6.9
1980	4,781	100.0	114	2.4	2,379	49.8	1,977	41.3	311	6.5
1982	5,167	100.0	189	3.7	2,673	51.7	2,089	40.4	216	4.2
1984	6,295	100.0	200	3.2	3,488	55.4	2,355	37.4	252	4.1
1986	5,818	100.0	330	5.7	3,728	64.1	1,645	28.3	115	2.0
1988	5,450	100.0	346	6.3	3,500	64.2	1,481	27.2	123	2.3
1990	6,106	100.0	353	5.8	3,851	63.1	1,778	29.1	124	2.0
1992	6,335	100.0	382	6.0	3,975	62.7	1,896	29.9	82	1.3
1994	9,737	100.0	477	4.9	5,392	55.4	3,327	34.2	541	5.6
1996	7,585	100.0	556	7.3	4,623	60.9	2,099	27.7	307	4.0
BACCALAUREATE AND HIGHER DEGREE PROGRAMS										
1978	1,919	100.0	109	5.7	1,278	66.6	522	27.2	10	0.5
1980	2,108	100.0	96	4.6	1,589	75.4	418	19.8	4	0.2
1982	2,254	100.0	177	7.9	1,672	74.2	404	17.9	1	0.0
1984	2,726	100.0	170	6.2	2,138	78.4	416	15.3	2	0.0
1986	2,962	100.0	282	9.5	2,379	80.3	299	10.1	2	0.1
1988	2,622	100.0	265	10.1	2,132	81.3	218	8.3	7	0.3
1990	2,571	100.0	290	11.3	2,057	80.0	217	8.4	7	0.3
1992	2,678	100.0	322	12.0	2,124	79.3	231	8.6	1	0.0
1994	3,444	100.0	380	11.0	2,709	78.7	353	10.2	2	0.1
1996	3,582	100.0	484	13.5	2,804	78.3	275	7.7	19	0.5
ASSOCIATE DEGREE PROGRAMS										
1978	1,622	100.0	8	0.5	486	30.0	989	61.0	139	7.5
1980	1,852	100.0	12	0.7	580	31.3	1,082	58.4	178	9.6
1982	2,146	100.0	7	0.3	768	35.8	1,240	57.8	131	6.1
1984	2,821	100.0	24	0.9	1,106	39.2	1,495	53.0	196	6.9
1986	2,317	100.0	39	1.7	1,101	47.5	1,093	47.2	84	3.6
1988	2,433	100.0	75	3.1	1,138	46.8	1,114	45.8	106	4.4
1990	3,109	100.0	60	1.9	1,508	48.5	1,427	45.9	114	3.7
1992	3,238	100.0	56	1.7	1,590	49.1	1,514	46.8	78	2.4
1994	3,950	100.0	73	1.8	2,001	50.7	1,760	44.6	116	2.9
1996	2,603	100.0	57	2.2	1,389	53.4	1,090	41.9	67	2.6
DIPLOMA PROGRAMS										
1978	916	100.0	14	1.5	211	23.0	532	58.1	159	17.4
1980	821	100.0	6	0.7	210	25.6	477	58.1	128	15.2
1982	767	100.0	5	0.7	233	30.4	445	58.0	84	10.9
1984	748	100.0	6	0.8	244	32.6	444	59.4	54	7.2
1986	539	100.0	9	1.7	248	46.0	253	46.9	29	5.4
1988	395	100.0	6	1.5	230	58.2	149	37.7	10	2.5
1990	426	100.0	3	0.7	286	67.1	134	31.5	3	0.7
1992	419	100.0	4	1.0	261	62.3	151	36.0	3	0.7
1994	486	100.0	8	1.6	317	65.2	152	31.3	9	1.9
1996	230	100.0	5	2.2	185	80.4	39	17.0	1	0.4
PN/VN PROGRAMS										
1978	N/A	N/A	N/A	N/A	N/A	N/A	N/A	N/A	N/A	N/A
1980	N/A	N/A	N/A	N/A	N/A	N/A	N/A	N/A	N/A	N/A
1982	N/A	N/A	N/A	N/A	N/A	N/A	N/A	N/A	N/A	N/A
1984	N/A	N/A	N/A	N/A	N/A	N/A	N/A	N/A	N/A	N/A
1986	N/A	N/A	N/A	N/A	N/A	N/A	N/A	N/A	N/A	N/A
1988	N/A	N/A	N/A	N/A	N/A	N/A	N/A	N/A	N/A	N/A
1990	N/A	N/A	N/A	N/A	N/A	N/A	N/A	N/A	N/A	N/A
1992	N/A	N/A	N/A	N/A	N/A	N/A	N/A	N/A	N/A	N/A
1994	1,857	100.0	16	0.9	365	19.7	1,062	57.2	414	22.3
1996	1,170	100.0	10	0.9	245	20.9	695	59.4	220	18.8

[1] Excludes American Samoa, Guam, Puerto Rico and the Virgin Islands.

48

Table 23
HIGHEST EARNED CREDENTIAL OF FULL-TIME FACULTY BY REGION, 1978-1996[1]

YEAR BY REGION[1]	TOTAL FULL-TIME FACULTY REPORTED		HIGHEST EARNED CREDENTIAL							
			DOCTORATE		MASTER'S		BACCALAUREATE		OTHER	
	Number	Percent	Number	Percent	Number	Percent	Number	Percent	Number	Percent
North Atlantic										
1978	5,498	100.0	273	5.0	3,508	63.8	1,514	27.5	203	3.7
1980	5,581	100.0	428	7.7	3,806	68.2	1,205	21.6	142	2.5
1982	5,333	100.0	493	9.2	3,798	71.2	953	17.9	89	1.7
1984	5,128	100.0	535	10.4	3,763	73.4	779	15.2	51	1.0
1986	4,980	100.0	705	14.2	3,731	74.9	513	10.3	31	0.6
1988	4,083	100.0	785	19.2	3,018	73.9	269	6.6	11	0.3
1990	4,181	100.0	919	22.0	3,018	72.2	226	5.4	18	0.4
1992	3,633	100.0	893	24.6	2,557	70.4	168	4.6	15	0.4
1994	4,251	100.0	905	21.3	2,798	65.8	476	11.2	72	1.7
1996	3,763	100.0	1,001	26.6	2,458	65.3	255	6.8	49	1.3
Midwest										
1978	6,245	100.0	295	4.7	3,406	54.5	2,296	36.8	248	4.0
1980	6,048	100.0	351	5.8	3,697	61.1	1,836	30.4	164	2.7
1982	5,979	100.0	428	7.2	3,936	65.8	1,522	25.4	93	1.6
1984	6,299	100.0	537	8.5	4,448	70.6	1,243	19.7	71	1.1
1986	4,930	100.0	485	9.8	3,690	74.9	702	14.2	53	1.0
1988	4,690	100.0	783	16.7	3,351	71.4	524	11.2	32	0.7
1990	4,660	100.0	894	19.2	3,322	71.3	424	9.1	20	0.4
1992	4,720	100.0	996	21.1	3,335	70.7	381	8.1	8	0.2
1994	5,539	100.0	1,137	20.5	3,619	65.3	673	12.2	110	2.0
1996	4,976	100.0	1,200	24.1	3,198	64.3	510	10.2	68	1.4
South										
1978	5,947	100.0	282	4.7	3,779	63.5	1,724	29.0	162	2.8
1980	6,209	100.0	378	6.1	4,361	70.2	1,364	22.0	106	1.7
1982	6,060	100.0	466	7.7	4,507	74.4	1,030	17.0	57	0.7
1984	6,295	100.0	676	10.7	4,709	74.8	863	13.7	47	0.7
1986	5,762	100.0	772	13.4	4,357	75.6	601	10.4	32	0.5
1988	5,625	100.0	1,056	18.8	4,213	74.9	341	6.1	15	0.3
1990	5,580	100.0	1,198	21.5	4,019	72.0	351	6.3	12	0.2
1992	5,739	100.0	1,305	22.7	3,977	69.3	441	7.7	16	0.3
1994	7,537	100.0	1,489	19.8	4,564	60.6	1,128	15.0	356	4.7
1996	6,630	100.0	1,491	22.5	4,067	61.3	749	11.3	323	4.9
West										
1978	2,527	100.0	212	8.4	1,944	76.8	331	13.2	40	1.6
1980	2,517	100.0	261	10.4	1,962	77.9	282	11.2	12	0.5
1982	2,370	100.0	270	11.4	1,844	77.8	246	10.4	10	0.4
1984	2,499	100.0	395	15.8	1,877	75.1	219	8.8	8	0.4
1986	2,306	100.0	442	19.2	1,703	73.9	153	6.6	8	0.4
1988	2,504	100.0	597	23.8	1,766	70.5	135	5.4	6	0.2
1990	2,235	100.0	554	24.8	1,531	68.5	146	6.5	4	0.2
1992	2,457	100.0	673	27.4	1,664	67.7	118	4.8	2	0.1
1994	2,634	100.0	691	26.2	1,626	61.7	285	10.8	32	1.2
1996	2,136	100.0	639	29.9	1,306	61.1	168	7.9	23	1.1

[1] Excludes American Samoa, Guam, Puerto Rico and the Virgin Islands.

Table 24
HIGHEST EARNED CREDENTIAL OF PART-TIME FACULTY BY REGION, 1996[1]

NLN REGION	TOTAL PART-TIME FACULTY REPORTED		HIGHEST EARNED CREDENTIAL							
			DOCTORATE		MASTER'S		BACCALAUREATE		OTHER	
	Number	Percent	Number	Percent	Number	Percent	Number	Percent	Number	Percent
All Regions	7,585	100.0	556	7.3	4,623	60.9	2,099	27.7	307	4.0
North Atlantic	1,925	100.0	161	8.4	1,315	68.3	374	19.4	75	3.9
Midwest	2,401	100.0	136	5.7	1,396	58.1	785	32.7	84	3.5
South	2,110	100.0	159	7.5	1,207	57.2	626	29.7	118	5.6
West	1,149	100.0	100	8.7	705	61.4	314	27.3	30	2.6

[1] Excludes American Samoa, Guam, Puerto Rico and the Virgin Islands

Table 25
FACULTY RANK OF FULL-TIME FACULTY BY REGION OF THE COUNTRY AND TYPE OF PROGRAM, 1996[1]

NLN REGION	TOTAL FULL-TIME FACULTY REPORTED		Professor		Associate Professor		Assistant Professor		Instructor		No Rank/Other Rank	
	Number	Percent	Number	Percent	Number	Percent	Number	Percent	Number	Percent	Number	Percent
ALL REPORTING PROGRAMS												
All Regions	17,443	100.0	1,815	10.4	3,213	18.4	4,881	28.0	5,982	34.3	1,552	8.9
North Atlantic	3,730	100.0	421	11.3	693	18.6	1,179	31.6	1,132	30.3	305	8.2
Midwest	4,961	100.0	422	8.5	1,016	20.5	1,385	27.9	1,565	31.5	573	11.6
South	6,609	100.0	514	7.8	1,113	16.8	1,881	28.5	2,606	39.4	495	7.5
West	2,143	100.0	458	21.4	391	18.2	436	20.3	679	31.7	179	8.4
BACCALAUREATE AND HIGHER DEGREE PROGRAMS												
All Regions	8,602	100.0	904	10.5	2,362	27.5	3,451	40.1	1,378	16.0	507	5.9
North Atlantic	1,813	100.0	174	9.6	504	27.8	781	43.1	254	14.0	100	5.5
Midwest	2,660	100.0	249	9.4	776	29.2	1,051	39.5	386	14.5	198	7.4
South	3,084	100.0	277	9.0	778	25.2	1,295	42.0	583	18.9	151	4.9
West	1,045	100.0	204	19.5	304	29.1	324	31.0	155	14.8	58	5.6
ASSOCIATE DEGREE PROGRAMS												
All Regions	5,470	100.0	797	14.6	781	14.3	1,281	23.4	2,022	37.0	589	10.8
North Atlantic	1,037	100.0	240	23.1	179	17.3	339	32.7	199	19.2	80	7.7
Midwest	1,456	100.0	144	9.9	225	15.5	296	20.3	596	40.9	195	13.4
South	2,217	100.0	211	9.5	318	14.3	555	25.0	906	40.9	227	10.2
West	760	100.0	202	26.6	59	7.8	91	12.0	321	42.2	87	11.4
DIPLOMA PROGRAMS												
All Regions	980	100.0	12	1.2	5	0.5	44	4.5	723	73.8	196	20.0
North Atlantic	489	100.0	0	0.0	2	0.4	23	4.7	397	81.2	67	13.7
Midwest	254	100.0	4	1.6	1	0.4	15	5.9	152	59.8	82	32.3
South	220	100.0	8	3.6	2	0.9	6	2.7	157	71.4	47	21.4
West	17	100.0	0	0.0	0	0.0	0	0.0	17	100.0	0	0.0
PN/VN NURSING PROGRAMS												
All Regions	2,391	100.0	102	4.3	65	2.7	105	4.4	1,859	77.7	260	10.9
North Atlantic	391	100.0	7	1.8	8	2.0	36	9.2	282	72.1	58	14.8
Midwest	591	100.0	25	4.2	14	2.4	23	3.9	431	72.9	98	16.6
South	1,088	100.0	18	1.7	15	1.4	25	2.3	960	88.2	70	6.4
West	321	100.0	52	16.2	28	8.7	21	6.5	186	57.9	34	10.6

[1] Excludes American Samoa, Guam, Puerto Rico and the Virgin Islands

50

Table 26

FACULTY RANK OF PART-TIME FACULTY BY REGION OF THE COUNTRY AND TYPE OF PROGRAM, 1996[1]

NLN REGION	TOTAL PART-TIME FACULTY REPORTED		Professor		Associate Professor		Assistant Professor		Instructor		No Rank/Other Rank	
	Number	Percent	Number	Percent	Number	Percent	Number	Percent	Number	Percent	Number	Percent
ALL REPORTING PROGRAMS												
All Regions	7,581	100.0	81	1.1	209	2.8	624	8.2	3,733	49.2	2,934	38.7
North Atlantic	1,918	100.0	12	0.6	57	3.0	194	10.1	863	45.0	792	41.3
Midwest	2,404	100.0	16	0.7	60	2.5	191	7.9	1,162	48.3	975	40.6
South	2,102	100.0	20	1.0	58	2.8	170	8.1	1,076	51.2	778	37.0
West	1,157	100.0	33	2.9	34	2.9	69	6.0	632	54.6	389	33.6
BACCALAUREATE AND HIGHER DEGREE PROGRAMS												
All Regions	3,595	100.0	41	1.1	136	3.8	474	13.2	1,422	39.6	1,522	42.3
North Atlantic	881	100.0	8	0.9	43	4.9	131	14.9	310	35.2	389	44.2
Midwest	1,132	100.0	14	1.2	35	3.1	139	12.3	471	41.6	473	41.8
South	1,009	100.0	9	0.9	38	3.8	151	15.0	406	40.2	405	40.1
West	573	100.0	10	1.7	20	3.5	53	9.2	235	41.0	255	44.5
ASSOCIATE DEGREE PROGRAMS												
All Regions	2,584	100.0	23	0.9	56	2.2	120	4.6	1,233	47.7	1,152	44.6
North Atlantic	597	100.0	3	0.5	13	2.2	46	7.7	211	35.3	324	54.3
Midwest	869	100.0	1	0.1	17	2.0	40	4.6	401	46.1	410	47.2
South	734	100.0	6	0.8	14	1.9	18	2.5	376	51.2	320	43.6
West	384	100.0	13	3.4	12	3.1	16	4.2	245	63.8	98	25.5
DIPLOMA PROGRAMS												
All Regions	228	100.0	1	0.4	2	0.9	6	2.6	158	69.3	61	26.8
North Atlantic	130	100.0	0	0.0	0	0.0	0	0.0	91	70.0	39	30.0
Midwest	55	100.0	0	0.0	2	3.6	6	10.9	33	60.0	14	25.5
South	43	100.0	1	2.3	0	0.0	0	0.0	34	79.1	8	18.6
West	0	0.0	0	0.0	0	0.0	0	0.0	0	0.0	0	0.0
PN/VN PROGRAMS												
All Regions	1,174	100.0	16	1.4	15	1.3	24	2.0	920	78.4	199	17.0
North Atlantic	310	100.0	1	0.3	1	0.3	17	5.5	251	81.0	40	12.9
Midwest	348	100.0	1	0.3	6	1.7	6	1.7	257	73.9	78	22.4
South	316	100.0	4	1.3	6	1.9	1	0.3	260	82.3	45	14.2
West	200	100.0	10	5.0	2	1.0	0	0.0	152	76.0	36	18.0

[1] Excludes American Samoa, Guam, Puerto Rico and the Virgin Islands

51

Table 27
LENGTH OF TIME AT INSTITUTION BY FACULTY RANK AND TYPE OF PROGRAM, 1996[1]

FACULTY RANK	TOTAL FULL-TIME FACULTY REPORTED		Less than 1 year		1-4 years		5-8 years		9-12 years		13-16 years		Longer than 16 years	
	Number	Percent	Number	Percent	Number	Percent	Number	Percent	Number	Percent	Number	Percent	Number	Percent
ALL REPORTING PROGRAMS														
Professor	1,803	100.0	50	2.8	159	8.8	235	13.0	258	14.3	332	18.4	769	42.7
Associate Professor	3,196	100.0	127	4.0	410	12.8	597	18.7	620	19.4	524	16.4	918	28.7
Assistant Professor	4,844	100.0	387	8.0	1,685	34.8	1,292	26.7	566	11.7	333	6.9	581	12.0
Instructor	5,931	100.0	613	10.3	2,316	39.0	1,269	21.4	527	8.9	456	7.7	750	12.6
No Rank/Other Rank	1,543	100.0	146	9.5	562	36.4	306	19.8	151	9.8	155	10.0	223	14.5
BACCALAUREATE AND HIGHER DEGREE PROGRAMS														
Professor	898	100.0	26	2.9	73	8.1	111	12.4	148	16.5	153	17.0	387	43.1
Associate Professor	2,351	100.0	108	4.6	352	15.0	398	16.9	455	19.4	373	15.9	665	28.3
Assistant Professor	3,425	100.0	299	8.7	1,206	35.2	825	24.1	401	11.7	242	7.1	452	13.2
Instructor	1,375	100.0	236	17.2	766	55.7	238	17.3	80	5.8	23	1.7	32	2.3
No Rank/Other Rank	505	100.0	66	13.1	251	49.7	83	16.4	40	7.9	31	6.1	34	6.7
ASSOCIATE DEGREE PROGRAMS														
Professor	791	100.0	16	2.0	66	8.3	114	14.4	89	11.3	159	20.1	347	43.9
Associate Professor	778	100.0	17	2.2	52	6.7	182	23.4	152	19.5	141	18.1	234	30.1
Assistant Professor	1,274	100.0	80	6.3	432	33.9	425	33.4	143	11.2	80	6.3	114	8.9
Instructor	2,009	100.0	187	9.3	774	38.5	408	20.3	189	9.4	190	9.5	261	13.0
No Rank/Other Rank	587	100.0	42	7.2	183	31.2	140	23.9	62	10.6	62	10.6	98	16.7
DIPLOMA PROGRAMS														
Professor	12	100.0	4	33.3	3	25.0	2	16.7	0	0.0	1	8.3	2	16.7
Associate Professor	4	100.0	0	0.0	0	0.0	2	50.0	0	0.0	0	0.0	2	50.0
Assistant Professor	42	100.0	0	0.0	3	7.1	15	35.7	12	28.6	5	11.9	7	16.7
Instructor	723	100.0	23	3.2	137	18.9	195	27.0	98	13.6	85	11.8	185	25.6
No Rank/Other Rank	196	100.0	18	9.2	49	25.0	27	13.8	26	13.3	27	13.8	49	25.0
PN/VN NURSING PROGRAMS														
Professor	102	100.0	4	3.9	17	16.7	8	7.8	21	20.6	19	18.6	33	32.4
Associate Professor	63	100.0	2	3.2	6	9.5	15	23.8	13	20.6	10	15.9	17	27.0
Assistant Professor	103	100.0	8	7.8	44	42.7	27	26.2	10	9.7	6	5.8	8	7.8
Instructor	1,824	100.0	167	9.2	639	35.0	428	23.5	160	8.8	158	8.7	272	14.9
No Rank/Other Rank	255	100.0	20	7.8	79	31.0	56	22.0	23	9.0	35	13.7	42	16.5

[1] Excludes American Samoa, Guam, Puerto Rico and the Virgin Islands

Table 28

SALARIES OF NURSING EDUCATION ADMINISTRATORS BY HIGHEST EARNED CREDENTIAL, AND TYPE OF PROGRAM, 1996[1]

HIGHEST EARNED CREDENTIAL	TOTAL ADMINISTRATORS REPORTED		SALARY RANGE									
	Number	Percent	Less than $15,000		$15,000-$29,999		$30,000-$44,999		$45,000-$59,999		$60,000-$74,999		$75,000 or More	
			Number	Percent	Number	Percent	Number	Percent	Number	Percent	Number	Percent	Number	Percent
ALL REPORTING PROGRAMS														
Total	1,662	100.0	2	0.1	19	1.1	372	22.4	648	39.0	401	24.1	220	13.2
Doctorate	689	100.0	0	0.0	0	0.0	46	6.7	216	31.3	239	34.7	188	27.3
Master's	825	100.0	0	0.0	7	0.8	222	26.9	404	49.0	161	19.5	31	3.8
Baccalaureate	120	100.0	2	0.7	9	7.5	84	70.0	24	20.0	1	0.8	0	0.0
Other	28	100.0	0	0.0	3	10.7	20	71.4	4	14.3	0	0.0	1	3.6
BACCALAUREATE AND HIGHER DEGREE PROGRAMS														
Total	530	100.0	0	0.0	1	0.2	42	7.9	146	27.5	171	32.3	170	32.1
Doctorate	492	100.0	0	0.0	0	0.0	28	5.7	131	26.6	166	33.7	167	33.9
Master's	36	100.0	0	0.0	1	2.8	14	38.9	14	38.9	5	13.9	2	5.6
Baccalaureate	0	0.0	0	0.0	0	0.0	0	0.0	0	0.0	0	0.0	0	0.0
Other	2	100.0	0	0.0	0	0.0	0	0.0	1	50.0	0	0.0	1	50.0
ASSOCIATE DEGREE PROGRAMS														
Total	544	100.0	0	0.0	5	0.9	116	21.3	264	48.5	128	23.5	31	5.7
Doctorate	146	100.0	0	0.0	0	0.0	14	9.6	67	45.9	50	34.2	15	10.3
Master's	394	100.0	0	0.0	4	1.0	99	25.1	197	50.0	78	19.8	16	4.1
Baccalaureate	3	100.0	0	0.0	1	33.3	2	66.7	0	0.0	0	0.0	0	0.0
Other	1	100.0	0	0.0	0	0.0	1	100.0	0	0.0	0	0.0	0	0.0
DIPLOMA PROGRAMS														
Total	70	100.0	0	0.0	0	0.0	2	2.9	21	30.0	34	48.6	13	18.6
Doctorate	15	100.0	0	0.0	0	0.0	0	0.0	2	13.3	8	53.3	5	33.3
Master's	55	100.0	0	0.0	0	0.0	2	3.6	19	34.5	26	47.3	8	14.5
Baccalaureate	0	0.0	0	0.0	0	0.0	0	0.0	0	0.0	0	0.0	0	0.0
Other	0	0.0	0	0.0	0	0.0	0	0.0	0	0.0	0	0.0	0	0.0
PN/VN PROGRAMS														
Total	518	100.0	2	0.4	13	2.5	212	40.9	217	41.9	68	13.1	6	1.2
Doctorate	36	100.0	0	0.0	0	0.0	4	11.1	16	44.4	15	41.7	1	2.8
Master's	340	100.0	0	0.0	2	0.6	107	31.5	174	51.2	52	15.3	5	1.5
Baccalaureate	117	100.0	2	1.7	8	6.8	82	70.1	24	20.5	1	0.9	0	0.0
Other	25	100.0	0	0.0	3	12.0	19	76.0	3	12.0	0	0.0	0	0.0

[1] Excludes American Samoa, Guam, Puerto Rico and the Virgin Islands

Table 29
SALARIES OF FULL-TIME FACULTY BY FACULTY RANK AND TYPE OF PROGRAM, 1996[1]

FACULTY RANK	TOTAL FULL-TIME FACULTY REPORTED		SALARY RANGE											
	Number	Percent	Less than $15,000		$15,000-$29,999		$30,000-$44,999		$45,000-$59,999		$60,000-$74,999		$75,000 or More	
			Number	Percent	Number	Percent	Number	Percent	Number	Percent	Number	Percent	Number	Percent
ALL REPORTING PROGRAMS														
Total	17,070	100.0	48	0.3	1,135	6.6	9,617	56.3	4,688	27.5	1,256	7.4	326	1.9
Professor	1,758	100.0	3	0.2	19	1.1	391	22.2	650	37.0	489	27.8	206	11.7
Associate Professor	3,172	100.0	0	0.0	22	0.7	1,191	37.5	1,455	45.9	431	13.6	73	2.3
Assistant Professor	4,791	100.0	5	0.1	242	5.1	3,334	69.6	1,041	21.7	147	3.1	22	0.5
Instructor	5,815	100.0	26	0.4	726	12.5	3,770	64.8	1,163	20.0	116	2.0	14	0.2
No Rank/Other Rank	1,534	100.0	14	0.9	126	8.2	931	60.7	379	24.7	73	4.8	11	0.7
BACCALAUREATE AND HIGHER DEGREE PROGRAMS														
Total	8,478	100.0	18	0.2	275	3.2	4,380	51.7	2,614	30.8	893	10.5	298	3.5
Professor	891	100.0	1	0.1	2	0.2	55	6.2	289	32.4	348	39.1	196	22.0
Associate Professor	2,339	100.0	0	0.0	5	0.2	718	30.7	1,170	50.0	377	16.1	69	2.9
Assistant Professor	3,402	100.0	1	0.0	99	2.9	2,275	66.9	881	25.9	125	3.7	21	0.6
Instructor	1,347	100.0	8	0.6	144	10.7	965	71.6	201	14.9	22	1.6	7	0.5
No Rank/Other Rank	499	100.0	8	1.6	25	5.0	367	73.5	73	14.6	21	4.2	5	1.0
ASSOCIATE DEGREE PROGRAMS														
Total	5,350	100.0	17	0.3	516	9.6	3,280	61.3	1,265	23.6	256	4.8	16	0.3
Professor	754	100.0	2	0.3	14	1.9	294	39.0	308	40.8	127	16.8	9	1.2
Associate Professor	766	100.0	0	0.0	15	2.0	437	57.0	260	33.9	50	6.5	4	0.5
Assistant Professor	1,251	100.0	4	0.3	130	10.4	968	77.4	126	10.1	22	1.8	1	0.1
Instructor	1,997	100.0	6	0.3	281	14.1	1,248	62.5	432	21.6	30	1.5	0	0.0
No Rank/Other Rank	582	100.0	5	0.9	76	13.1	333	57.2	139	23.9	27	4.6	2	0.3
DIPLOMA PROGRAMS														
Total	931	100.0	1	0.1	16	1.7	517	55.5	335	36.0	53	5.7	9	1.0
Professor	11	100.0	0	0.0	0	0.0	8	72.7	3	27.3	0	0.0	0	0.0
Associate Professor	3	100.0	0	0.0	0	0.0	1	33.3	1	33.3	1	33.3	0	0.0
Assistant Professor	38	100.0	0	0.0	0	0.0	19	50.0	19	50.0	0	0.0	0	0.0
Instructor	684	100.0	1	0.1	13	1.9	389	56.9	234	34.2	40	5.8	7	1.0
No Rank/Other Rank	195	100.0	0	0.0	3	1.5	100	51.3	78	40.0	12	6.2	2	1.0
PN/VN PROGRAMS														
Total	2,311	100.0	12	0.5	328	14.2	1,440	62.3	474	20.5	54	2.3	3	0.1
Professor	102	100.0	0	0.0	3	2.9	34	33.3	50	49.0	14	13.7	1	1.0
Associate Professor	64	100.0	0	0.0	2	3.1	35	54.7	24	37.5	3	4.7	0	0.0
Assistant Professor	100	100.0	0	0.0	13	13.0	72	72.0	15	15.0	0	0.0	0	0.0
Instructor	1,787	100.0	11	0.6	288	16.1	1,168	65.4	296	16.6	24	1.3	0	0.0
No Rank/Other Rank	258	100.0	1	0.4	22	8.5	131	50.8	89	34.5	13	5.0	2	0.8

[1] Excludes American Samoa, Guam, Puerto Rico and the Virgin Islands

Table 30
SALARIES OF PART-TIME FACULTY BY FACULTY RANK AND TYPE OF PROGRAM, 1996[1]

FACULTY RANK	TOTAL PART-TIME FACULTY REPORTED		SALARY RANGE											
	Number	Percent	Less than $15,000		$15,000-$29,999		$30,000-$44,999		$45,000-$59,999		$60,000-$74,999		$75,000 or More	
			Number	Percent	Number	Percent	Number	Percent	Number	Percent	Number	Percent	Number	Percent
ALL REPORTING PROGRAMS														
Total	7,291	100.0	4,720	64.7	1,663	22.8	639	8.8	211	2.9	47	0.6	11	0.2
Professor	71	100.0	11	15.5	16	22.5	12	16.9	20	28.2	8	11.3	4	5.6
Associate Professor	200	100.0	72	36.0	40	20.0	30	15.0	37	18.5	18	9.0	3	1.5
Assistant Professor	586	100.0	231	39.4	191	32.6	110	18.8	42	7.2	10	1.7	2	0.3
Instructor	3,620	100.0	2,262	62.5	960	26.5	314	8.7	77	2.1	6	0.2	1	0.0
No Rank/Other Rank	2,814	100.0	2,144	76.2	456	16.2	173	6.1	35	1.2	5	0.2	1	0.0
BACCALAUREATE AND HIGHER DEGREE PROGRAMS														
Total	3,469	100.0	2,091	60.3	799	23.0	376	10.8	157	4.5	35	1.0	11	0.3
Professor	38	100.0	2	5.3	4	10.5	7	18.4	13	34.2	8	21.1	4	10.5
Associate Professor	127	100.0	39	30.7	23	18.1	19	15.0	31	24.4	12	9.4	3	2.4
Assistant Professor	441	100.0	144	32.7	148	33.6	98	22.2	39	8.8	10	2.3	2	0.5
Instructor	1,387	100.0	810	58.4	398	28.7	130	9.4	46	3.3	2	0.1	1	0.1
No Rank/Other Rank	1,476	100.0	1,096	74.3	226	15.3	122	8.3	28	1.9	3	0.2	1	0.1
ASSOCIATE DEGREE PROGRAMS														
Total	2,474	100	1,929	78.0	412	16.7	105	4.2	19	0.8	9	0.4	0	0.0
Professor	18	100	4	22.2	8	44.4	3	16.7	3	16.7	0	0.0	0	0.0
Associate Professor	56	100	24	42.9	14	25.0	10	17.9	2	3.6	6	10.7	0	0.0
Assistant Professor	120	100	70	58.3	37	30.8	10	8.3	3	2.5	0	0.0	0	0.0
Instructor	1,202	100	933	77.6	211	17.6	48	4.0	7	0.6	3	0.2	0	0.0
No Rank/Other Rank	1,078	100	898	83.3	142	13.2	34	3.2	4	0.4	0	0.0	0	0.0
DIPLOMA PROGRAMS														
Total	224	100.0	23	10.3	125	55.8	55	24.6	18	8.0	3	1.3	0	0.0
Professor	1	100.0	0	0.0	0	0.0	1	100.0	0	0.0	0	0.0	0	0.0
Associate Professor	2	100.0	0	0.0	2	100.0	0	0.0	0	0.0	0	0.0	0	0.0
Assistant Professor	6	100.0	0	0.0	5	83.3	1	16.7	0	0.0	0	0.0	0	0.0
Instructor	154	100.0	13	8.4	70	45.5	52	33.8	18	11.7	1	0.6	0	0.0
No Rank/Other Rank	61	100.0	10	16.4	48	78.7	1	1.6	0	0.0	2	3.3	0	0.0
PN/VN PROGRAMS														
Total	1,124	100.0	677	60.2	327	29.1	103	9.2	17	1.5	0	0.0	0	0.0
Professor	14	100.0	5	35.7	4	28.6	1	7.1	4	28.6	0	0.0	0	0.0
Associate Professor	15	100.0	9	60.0	1	6.7	1	6.7	4	26.7	0	0.0	0	0.0
Assistant Professor	19	100.0	17	89.5	1	5.3	1	5.3	0	0.0	0	0.0	0	0.0
Instructor	877	100.0	506	57.7	281	32.0	84	9.6	6	0.7	0	0.0	0	0.0
No Rank/Other Rank	199	100.0	140	70.4	40	20.1	16	8.0	3	1.5	0	0.0	0	0.0

[1] Excludes American Samoa, Guam, Puerto Rico and the Virgin Islands

Table 31
SALARIES OF FULL-TIME FACULTY BY FACULTY RANK AND REGION, 1996[1]

FACULTY RANK	TOTAL FULL-TIME FACULTY REPORTED		SALARY RANGE											
	Number	Percent	Less than $15,000		$15,000-$29,999		$30,000-$44,999		$45,000-$59,999		$60,000-$74,999		$75,000 or More	
			Number	Percent	Number	Percent	Number	Percent	Number	Percent	Number	Percent	Number	Percent
ALL REGIONS														
Total	17,070	100.0	48	0.3	1,135	6.6	9,617	56.3	4,688	27.5	1,256	7.4	326	1.9
Professor	1,758	100.0	3	0.2	19	1.1	391	22.2	650	37.0	489	27.8	206	11.7
Associate Professor	3,172	100.0	0	0.0	22	0.7	1,191	37.5	1,455	45.9	431	13.6	73	2.3
Assistant Professor	4,791	100.0	5	0.1	242	5.1	3,334	69.6	1,041	21.7	147	3.1	22	0.5
Instructor	5,815	100.0	26	0.4	726	12.5	3,770	64.8	1,163	20.0	116	2.0	14	0.2
No Rank/Other Rank	1,534	100.0	14	0.9	126	8.2	931	60.7	379	24.7	73	4.8	11	0.7
NORTH ATLANTIC														
Total	3,639	100.0	6	0.2	106	2.9	1,891	52.0	1,219	33.5	343	9.4	74	2.0
Professor	407	100.0	1	0.2	0	0.0	114	28.0	136	33.4	114	28.0	42	10.3
Associate Professor	684	100.0	0	0.0	2	0.3	205	30.0	349	51.0	114	16.7	14	2.0
Assistant Professor	1,144	100.0	3	0.3	23	2.0	735	64.2	323	28.2	51	4.5	9	0.8
Instructor	1,104	100.0	1	0.1	59	5.3	707	64.0	291	26.4	42	3.8	4	0.4
No Rank/Other Rank	300	100.0	1	0.3	22	7.3	130	43.3	120	40.0	22	7.3	5	1.7
MIDWEST														
Total	4,911	100.0	13	0.3	391	8.0	2,826	57.5	1,278	26.0	311	6.3	92	1.9
Professor	418	100.0	0	0.0	3	0.7	69	16.5	177	42.3	108	25.8	61	14.6
Associate Professor	1,005	100.0	0	0.0	12	1.2	400	39.8	437	43.5	132	13.1	24	2.4
Assistant Professor	1,367	100.0	1	0.1	84	6.1	1,041	76.2	202	14.8	36	2.6	3	0.2
Instructor	1,553	100.0	11	0.7	241	15.5	987	63.6	305	19.6	8	0.5	1	0.1
No Rank/Other Rank	568	100.0	1	0.2	51	9.0	329	57.9	157	27.6	27	4.8	3	0.5
SOUTH														
Total	6,422	100.0	19	0.3	543	8.5	4,028	62.7	1,413	22.0	318	5.0	101	1.6
Professor	504	100.0	1	0.2	9	1.8	167	33.1	161	31.9	103	20.4	63	12.5
Associate Professor	1,096	100.0	0	0.0	4	0.4	466	42.5	460	42.0	138	12.6	28	2.6
Assistant Professor	1,852	100.0	0	0.0	126	6.8	1,306	70.5	375	20.2	37	2.0	8	0.4
Instructor	2,483	100.0	11	0.4	362	14.6	1,723	69.4	357	14.4	28	1.1	2	0.1
No Rank/Other Rank	487	100.0	7	1.4	42	8.6	366	75.2	60	12.3	12	2.5	0	0.0
WEST														
Total	2,098	100.0	10	0.5	95	4.5	872	41.6	778	37.1	284	13.5	59	2.8
Professor	429	100.0	1	0.2	7	1.6	41	9.6	176	41.0	164	38.2	40	9.3
Associate Professor	387	100.0	0	0.0	4	1.0	120	31.0	209	54.0	47	12.1	7	1.8
Assistant Professor	428	100.0	1	0.2	9	2.1	252	58.9	141	32.9	23	5.4	2	0.5
Instructor	675	100.0	3	0.4	64	9.5	353	52.3	210	31.1	38	5.6	7	1.0
No Rank/Other Rank	179	100.0	5	2.8	11	6.1	106	59.2	42	23.5	12	6.7	3	1.7

[1] Excludes American Samoa, Guam, Puerto Rico and the Virgin Islands

Table 32
SALARIES OF FULL-TIME BACCALAUREATE AND HIGHER DEGREE FACULTY BY FACULTY RANK AND REGION, 1996[1]

FACULTY RANK	TOTAL FULL-TIME FACULTY REPORTED		SALARY RANGE											
	Number	Percent	Less than $15,000		$15,000-$29,999		$30,000-$44,999		$45,000-$59,999		$60,000-$74,999		$75,000 or More	
			Number	Percent	Number	Percent	Number	Percent	Number	Percent	Number	Percent	Number	Percent
ALL REGIONS														
Total	8,478	100.0	18	0.2	275	3.2	4,380	51.7	2,614	30.8	893	10.5	298	3.5
Professor	891	100.0	1	0.1	2	0.2	55	6.2	289	32.4	348	39.1	196	22.0
Associate Professor	2,339	100.0	0	0.0	5	0.2	718	30.7	1,170	50.0	377	16.1	69	2.9
Assistant Professor	3,402	100.0	1	0.0	99	2.9	2,275	66.9	881	25.9	125	3.7	21	0.6
Instructor	1,347	100.0	8	0.6	144	10.7	965	71.6	201	14.9	22	1.6	7	0.5
No Rank/Other Rank	499	100.0	8	1.6	25	5.0	367	73.5	73	14.6	21	4.2	5	1.0
NORTH ATLANTIC														
Total	1,782	100.0	1	0.1	28	1.6	835	46.9	615	34.5	238	13.4	65	3.6
Professor	172	100.0	0	0.0	0	0.0	9	5.2	43	25.0	80	46.5	40	23.3
Associate Professor	499	100.0	0	0.0	0	0.0	129	25.9	260	52.1	99	19.8	11	2.2
Assistant Professor	761	100.0	0	0.0	10	1.3	447	58.7	255	33.5	41	5.4	8	1.1
Instructor	253	100.0	0	0.0	18	7.1	192	75.9	31	12.3	9	3.6	3	1.2
No Rank/Other Rank	97	100.0	1	1.0	0	0.0	58	59.8	26	26.8	9	9.3	3	3.1
MIDWEST														
Total	2,623	100.0	2	0.1	109	4.2	1,529	58.3	679	25.9	217	8.3	87	3.3
Professor	245	100.0	0	0.0	0	0.0	27	11.0	91	37.1	68	27.8	59	24.1
Associate Professor	766	100.0	0	0.0	3	0.4	277	36.2	356	46.5	107	14.0	23	3.0
Assistant Professor	1,035	100.0	0	0.0	41	4.0	782	75.6	175	16.9	34	3.3	3	0.3
Instructor	379	100.0	2	0.5	53	14.0	293	77.3	29	7.7	1	0.3	1	0.3
No Rank/Other Rank	198	100.0	0	0.0	12	6.1	150	75.8	28	14.1	7	3.5	1	0.5
SOUTH														
Total	3,035	100.0	14	0.5	124	4.1	1,610	53.0	923	30.4	264	8.7	100	3.3
Professor	273	100.0	1	0.4	2	0.7	16	5.9	101	37.0	91	33.3	62	22.7
Associate Professor	771	100.0	0	0.0	0	0.0	232	30.1	380	49.3	131	17.0	28	3.6
Assistant Professor	1,284	100.0	0	0.0	47	3.7	862	67.1	335	26.1	32	2.5	8	0.6
Instructor	561	100.0	6	1.1	64	11.4	386	68.8	97	17.3	6	1.1	2	0.4
No Rank/Other Rank	146	100.0	7	4.8	11	7.5	114	78.1	10	6.8	4	2.7	0	0.0
WEST														
Total	1,038	100.0	1	0.1	14	1.3	406	39.1	397	38.2	174	16.8	46	4.4
Professor	201	100.0	0	0.0	0	0.0	3	1.5	54	26.9	109	54.2	35	17.4
Associate Professor	303	100.0	0	0.0	2	0.7	80	26.4	174	57.4	40	13.2	7	2.3
Assistant Professor	322	100.0	1	0.3	1	0.3	184	57.1	116	36.0	18	5.6	2	0.6
Instructor	154	100.0	0	0.0	9	5.8	94	61.0	44	28.6	6	3.9	1	0.6
No Rank/Other Rank	58	100.0	0	0.0	2	3.4	45	77.6	9	15.5	1	1.7	1	1.7

[1] Excludes American Samoa, Guam, Puerto Rico and the Virgin Islands

Table 33

SALARIES OF FULL-TIME ASSOCIATE DEGREE FACULTY BY FACULTY RANK AND REGION, 1996[1]

FACULTY RANK	TOTAL FULL-TIME FACULTY REPORTED		SALARY RANGE									
	Number	Percent	Less than $15,000		$15,000-$29,999		$30,000-$44,999		$45,000-$59,999		$60,000-$74,999		$75,000 or More
			Number	Percent	Number	Percent	Number	Percent	Number	Percent	Number	Percent	Number	Percent
ALL REGIONS														
Total	5,350	100.0	17	0.3	516	9.6	3,280	61.3	1,265	23.6	256	4.8	16	0.3
Professor	754	100.0	2	0.3	14	1.9	294	39.0	308	40.8	127	16.8	9	1.2
Associate Professor	766	100.0	0	0.0	15	2.0	437	57.0	260	33.9	50	6.5	4	0.5
Assistant Professor	1,251	100.0	4	0.3	130	10.4	968	77.4	126	10.1	22	1.8	1	0.1
Instructor	1,997	100.0	6	0.3	281	14.1	1,248	62.5	432	21.6	30	1.5	0	0.0
No Rank/Other Rank	582	100.0	5	0.9	76	13.1	333	57.2	139	23.9	27	4.6	2	0.3
NORTH ATLANTIC														
Total	991	100.0	4	0.4	41	4.1	593	59.8	290	29.3	57	5.8	6	0.6
Professor	228	100.0	1	0.4	0	0.0	105	46.1	89	39.0	31	13.6	2	0.9
Associate Professor	175	100.0	0	0.0	2	1.1	73	41.7	83	47.4	14	8.0	3	1.7
Assistant Professor	324	100.0	3	0.9	11	3.4	252	77.8	47	14.5	10	3.1	1	0.3
Instructor	186	100.0	0	0.0	14	7.5	126	67.7	46	24.7	0	0.0	0	0.0
No Rank/Other Rank	78	100.0	0	0.0	14	17.9	37	47.4	25	32.1	2	2.6	0	0.0
MIDWEST														
Total	1,447	100.0	2	0.1	187	12.9	766	52.9	404	27.9	84	5.8	4	0.3
Professor	144	100.0	0	0.0	3	2.1	26	18.1	74	51.4	39	27.1	2	1.4
Associate Professor	224	100.0	0	0.0	8	3.6	113	50.4	77	34.4	25	11.2	1	0.4
Assistant Professor	294	100.0	1	0.3	36	12.2	232	78.9	23	7.8	2	0.7	0	0.0
Instructor	595	100.0	1	0.2	108	18.2	318	53.4	161	27.1	7	1.2	0	0.0
No Rank/Other Rank	190	100.0	0	0.0	32	16.8	77	40.5	69	36.3	11	5.8	1	0.5
SOUTH														
Total	2,184	100.0	2	0.1	248	11.4	1,604	73.4	301	13.8	28	1.3	1	0.0
Professor	206	100.0	0	0.0	7	3.4	134	65.0	54	26.2	10	4.9	1	0.5
Associate Professor	310	100.0	0	0.0	4	1.3	224	72.3	76	24.5	6	1.9	0	0.0
Assistant Professor	543	100.0	0	0.0	79	14.5	424	78.1	35	6.4	5	0.9	0	0.0
Instructor	898	100.0	2	0.2	133	14.8	642	71.5	118	13.1	3	0.3	0	0.0
No Rank/Other Rank	227	100.0	0	0.0	25	11.0	180	79.3	18	7.9	4	1.8	0	0.0
WEST														
Total	728	100.0	9	1.2	40	5.5	317	43.5	270	37.1	87	12.0	5	0.7
Professor	176	100.0	1	0.6	4	2.3	29	16.5	91	51.7	47	26.7	4	2.3
Associate Professor	57	100.0	0	0.0	1	1.8	27	47.4	24	42.1	5	8.8	0	0.0
Assistant Professor	90	100.0	0	0.0	4	4.4	60	66.7	21	23.3	5	5.6	0	0.0
Instructor	318	100.0	3	0.9	26	8.2	162	50.9	107	33.6	20	6.3	0	0.0
No Rank/Other Rank	87	100.0	5	5.7	5	5.7	39	44.8	27	31.0	10	11.5	1	1.1

[1] Excludes American Samoa, Guam, Puerto Rico and the Virgin Islands

Table 34
SALARIES OF FULL-TIME DIPLOMA FACULTY BY FACULTY RANK AND REGION, 1996[1]

FACULTY RANK	TOTAL FULL-TIME FACULTY REPORTED		SALARY RANGE											
	Number	Percent	Less than $15,000		$15,000-$29,999		$30,000-$44,999		$45,000-$59,999		$60,000-$74,999		$75,000 or More	
			Number	Percent	Number	Percent	Number	Percent	Number	Percent	Number	Percent	Number	Percent
ALL REGIONS														
Total	931	100.0	1	0.1	16	1.7	517	55.5	335	36.0	53	5.7	9	1.0
Professor	11	100.0	0	0.0	0	0.0	8	72.7	3	27.3	0	0.0	0	0.0
Associate Professor	3	100.0	0	0.0	0	0.0	1	33.3	1	33.3	1	33.3	0	0.0
Assistant Professor	38	100.0	0	0.0	0	0.0	19	50.0	19	50.0	0	0.0	0	0.0
Instructor	684	100.0	1	0.1	13	1.9	389	56.9	234	34.2	40	5.8	7	1.0
No Rank/Other Rank	195	100.0	0	0.0	3	1.5	100	51.3	78	40.0	12	6.2	2	1.0
NORTH ATLANTIC														
TOTAL	479	100.0	1	0.2	10	2.1	219	45.7	211	44.1	35	7.3	3	0.6
Professor	0	0.0	0	0.0	0	0.0	0	0.0	0	0.0	0	0.0	0	0.0
Associate Professor	2	100.0	0	0.0	0	0.0	0	0.0	1	50.0	1	50.0	0	0.0
Assistant Professor	23	100.0	0	0.0	0	0.0	6	26.1	17	73.9	0	0.0	0	0.0
Instructor	387	100.0	1	0.3	7	1.8	200	51.7	153	39.5	25	6.5	1	0.3
No Rank/Other Rank	67	100.0	0	0.0	3	4.5	13	19.4	40	59.7	9	13.4	2	3.0
MIDWEST														
Total	254	100.0	0	0.0	6	2.4	186	73.2	61	24.0	1	0.4	0	0.0
Professor	4	100.0	0	0.0	0	0.0	2	50.0	2	50.0	0	0.0	0	0.0
Associate Professor	1	100.0	0	0.0	0	0.0	1	100.0	0	0.0	0	0.0	0	0.0
Assistant Professor	15	100.0	0	0.0	0	0.0	13	86.7	2	13.3	0	0.0	0	0.0
Instructor	152	100.0	0	0.0	6	3.9	108	71.1	38	25.0	0	0.0	0	0.0
No Rank/Other Rank	82	100.0	0	0.0	0	0.0	62	75.6	19	23.2	1	1.2	0	0.0
SOUTH														
Total	181	100.0	0	0.0	0	0.0	112	61.9	63	34.8	6	3.3	0	0.0
Professor	7	100.0	0	0.0	0	0.0	6	85.7	1	14.3	0	0.0	0	0.0
Associate Professor	0	0.0	0	0.0	0	0.0	0	0.0	0	0.0	0	0.0	0	0.0
Assistant Professor	0	0.0	0	0.0	0	0.0	0	0.0	0	0.0	0	0.0	0	0.0
Instructor	128	100.0	0	0.0	0	0.0	81	63.3	43	33.6	4	3.1	0	0.0
No Rank/Other Rank	46	100.0	0	0.0	0	0.0	25	54.3	19	41.3	2	4.3	0	0.0
WEST														
Total	17	100.0	0	0.0	0	0.0	0	0.0	0	0.0	11	64.7	6	35.3
Professor	0	0.0	0	0.0	0	0.0	0	0.0	0	0.0	0	0.0	0	0.0
Associate Professor	0	0.0	0	0.0	0	0.0	0	0.0	0	0.0	0	0.0	0	0.0
Assistant Professor	0	0.0	0	0.0	0	0.0	0	0.0	0	0.0	0	0.0	0	0.0
Instructor	17	100.0	0	0.0	0	0.0	0	0.0	0	0.0	11	64.7	6	35.3
No Rank/Other Rank	0	0.0	0	0.0	0	0.0	0	0.0	0	0.0	0	0.0	0	0.0

[1] Excludes American Samoa, Guam, Puerto Rico and the Virgin Islands

Table 35
SALARIES OF FULL-TIME PRACTICAL/VOCATIONAL NURSING FACULTY BY FACULTY RANK AND REGION, 1996[1]

FACULTY RANK	TOTAL FULL-TIME FACULTY REPORTED		SALARY RANGE											
	Number	Percent	Less than $15,000		$15,000-$29,999		$30,000-$44,999		$45,000-$59,999		$60,000-$74,999		$75,000 or More	
			Number	Percent	Number	Percent	Number	Percent	Number	Percent	Number	Percent	Number	Percent
Total	2,311	100.0	12	0.5	328	14.2	1,440	62.3	474	20.5	54	2.3	3	0.1
Professor	102	100.0	0	0.0	3	2.9	34	33.3	50	49.0	14	13.7	1	1.0
Associate Professor	64	100.0	0	0.0	2	3.1	35	54.7	24	37.5	3	4.7	0	0.0
Assistant Professor	100	100.0	0	0.0	13	13.0	72	72.0	15	15.0	0	0.0	0	0.0
Instructor	1,787	100.0	11	0.6	288	16.1	1,168	65.4	296	16.6	24	1.3	0	0.0
No Rank/Other Rank	258	100.0	1	0.4	22	8.5	131	50.8	89	34.5	13	5.0	2	0.8
NORTH ATLANTIC														
Total	387	100.0	0	0.0	27	7.0	244	63.0	103	26.6	13	3.4	0	0.0
Professor	7	100.0	0	0.0	0	0.0	0	0.0	4	57.1	3	42.9	0	0.0
Associate Professor	8	100.0	0	0.0	0	0.0	3	37.5	5	62.5	0	0.0	0	0.0
Assistant Professor	36	100.0	0	0.0	2	5.6	30	83.3	4	11.1	0	0.0	0	0.0
Instructor	278	100.0	0	0.0	20	7.2	189	68.0	61	21.9	8	2.9	0	0.0
No Rank/Other Rank	58	100.0	0	0.0	5	8.6	22	37.9	29	50.0	2	3.4	0	0.0
MIDWEST														
Total	587	100.0	9	1.5	89	15.2	345	58.8	134	22.8	9	1.5	1	0.2
Professor	25	100.0	0	0.0	0	0.0	14	56.0	10	40.0	1	4.0	0	0.0
Associate Professor	14	100.0	0	0.0	1	7.1	9	64.3	4	28.6	0	0.0	0	0.0
Assistant Professor	23	100.0	0	0.0	7	30.4	14	60.9	2	8.7	0	0.0	0	0.0
Instructor	427	100.0	8	1.9	74	17.3	268	62.8	77	18.0	0	0.0	0	0.0
No Rank/Other Rank	98	100.0	1	1.0	7	7.1	40	40.8	41	41.8	8	8.2	1	1.0
SOUTH														
Total	1,022	100.0	3	0.3	171	16.7	702	68.7	126	12.3	20	2.0	0	0.0
Professor	18	100.0	0	0.0	0	0.0	11	61.1	5	27.8	2	11.1	0	0.0
Associate Professor	15	100.0	0	0.0	0	0.0	10	66.7	4	26.7	1	6.7	0	0.0
Assistant Professor	25	100.0	0	0.0	0	0.0	20	80.0	5	20.0	0	0.0	0	0.0
Instructor	896	100.0	3	0.3	165	18.4	614	68.5	99	11.0	15	1.7	0	0.0
No Rank/Other Rank	68	100.0	0	0.0	6	8.8	47	69.1	13	19.1	2	2.9	0	0.0
WEST														
Total	315	100.0	0	0.0	41	13.0	149	47.3	111	35.2	12	3.8	2	0.6
Professor	52	100.0	0	0.0	3	5.8	9	17.3	31	59.6	8	15.4	1	1.9
Associate Professor	27	100.0	0	0.0	1	3.7	13	48.1	11	40.7	2	7.4	0	0.0
Assistant Professor	16	100.0	0	0.0	4	25.0	8	50.0	4	25.0	0	0.0	0	0.0
Instructor	186	100.0	0	0.0	29	15.6	97	52.2	59	31.7	1	0.5	0	0.0
No Rank/Other Rank	34	100.0	0	0.0	4	11.8	22	64.7	6	17.6	1	2.9	1	2.9

[1] Excludes American Samoa, Guam, Puerto Rico and the Virgin Islands